You, But Thinner:

Get Healthy & Be Happy NOW!

Contents

1- Introduction 2

2 - Your Nutrition 3

    Vegetables..4

    Fruits 13

    Whole Grains...17

    Dairy and Dairy Substitutes....................23

    Lean Proteins 26

    Fats and Oils..26

2.1 - The Importance of Nutrition.................27

    How Much and When to Eat....................30

    Choosing Good Foods While Eating Out 32

    How Good Food Benefits Your Body Inside And Out 34

2.2 - Good Foods 36

    Why You Should Be Limiting Sugars and Carbohydrates..36

        Low-Glycemic Sugars 37

        Artificial Sweeteners 38

        Sugar Alcohols..41

    How to Use "Good" Sugar In Cooking.......42

    Adding Whole Grains to Your Diet...........43

    Dealing with Food Allergies 45

        Peanut Allergies 45

Lactose Sensitivity and Milk Allergies 45

Gluten Allergies 46

Soy Allergies 47

2.3 - Foods That Have a Negative Impact On Your
Health.. 47

Frozen Meals 48

Candy 49

Canned Foods 50

Energy Drinks and Sports Drinks 50

"Healthy" Fast Food Meals 51

2.4 - Supplementing Your Diet 52

2.5 - Juicing and Green Smoothies 54

2.6 - Food Measurements – What Is An Appropriate
Portion Size? 55

2.7 - Meal Planning 58

2.8 - Food Preparation/Storage 60

Deep Freezing and Dehydrating Fresh Food 60

2.9 - Food Logs 62

3 - Exercise 63

How to Start an Exercise Program 64

Building a Walking Regimen 64

Building a Running Routine 65

Other Workout Methods for Starting Slow and Building Strong...66

Calculating Calories Burned For Optimum Weight Loss 67

Exercising Safely...68

3.1 - The Importance of Exercise 69

3.2 - Effective Exercise 71

Body Toning and Strengthening Exercises.................72

Strength Training For Beginners 72

Play Games with Your Children...............................75

3.3 - Ineffective Exercise 76

Exercises That Do Not Benefit Weight Loss 76

Exercises That Can Hurt Your Physical Well-Being....77

Exercises That Can Exacerbate Current Physical Conditions 79

Alternative Exercises for Weight Loss......................80

3.4 - Fitness Challenges......................................81

3.5 - Sports Wear Accessories to Add To Your Routine 83

4 - Accomplishing your Weight Loss Goals 86

Keeping Realistic Goals 86

Write Down Your Goals..87

Visualize Your Goals 88

Pick Yourself Up 88

Aim For the 10% Goal 89

Starting Small Leads to Something Big 89

Dealing with Setbacks 90

Measure Your Progress...90

Find A Weight Loss Partner Or Gym Buddy 91

Sticking With Your Plan For The Long Haul...............93

4.1 - Maintaining Your Progress.....................................94

1- Introduction

Dieting has become a term that gains negative media attention everywhere the word is said. Friends and family have disputes over different diets, and medical doctors go head to head with which diets are truly the best and how to lose weight for life. How do you know what to do, when everything tells you something different or contradicting? Health and nutrition has numerous benefits that go far beyond the typical goal of looking slim on the outside. But instead, when you eat right and exercise your body is nurtured from the inside out. You gain strength in your muscles, your body functions at optimum efficiency, and your brain even gets a boost.

In fact, exercise and proper diet can prevent most common diseases and health complications that Americans face today. Alzheimer's can be slowed down by walking at least six miles per week. Intense exercise boosts your brains power, and that is a scientific fact. Once you make an effort to change your lifestyle, your body adapts and responds to those changes.

A balanced diet with adequate protein, carbohydrates, healthy fats, and calories, will result in shedding pounds faster than if you skimped on some nutrients your body needs. Plus, with a healthy lifestyle change you won't need to take additional vitamins or minerals. You will be consuming all of the necessary vitamins through fruits, vegetables, and grains.

Another benefit of adhering to a healthy lifestyle plan is muscle function. When you eat poorly and don't exercise enough, muscles begin to lose their strength and elasticity. Your body becomes fattier, which puts you at risk for organ failure and heart disease. Developing lean muscle tissue will not only help you burn fat faster, but keep you going even during rest periods.

The core principles you will need for effective weight loss are motivation, nutrition, exercise, and plenty of sleep. Most people are overtired, malnourished, and in desperate need of a lifestyle change. If you are ready to be jolted out of your rundown and boring routine, then this is what you need. Weight gain doesn't happen overnight, so weight loss shouldn't either. You don't need expensive pills or crazy diets to help you reach your goals either. With dedication anything is possible.

This book will provide you with accurate and solid information to help you lose weight without starving. With a plan and information in front of you, it will be easy to reach your goals. If you need to lose 5 pounds or 50 pounds, you will get there in a timely manner without the risks associated with complicated and dangerous diets, fads, and pills. With the right information and goals you will find that losing weight doesn't have to be as hard as everyone makes it out to be. Making a healthy lifestyle change is a great way to see your goals flourish and come to life.

2 - Your Nutrition

So one of the first things that come to mind when weight loss is involved is "going on a diet". This will usually make people discouraged to continue because they believe that they will have to start eating salads and skipping out on all of the great tasting food that they are used to. This could not be anything but far from the truth. Instead of going on a diet, there can be changes to the diet which can have a positive impact on losing weight. More importantly, proper nutrition is something that should be implemented to help get the body on the right track to feeling healthy and losing weight.

A balanced diet defined by the USDA is a balance of fruits, vegetables, grains, protein, dairy, and a small amount of fat and sugars. But what does all of that mean? What if you have special dietary needs that limit your consumption of certain foods?

Vegetables

Starting with vegetables should be the core foundation of your new diet. Green leafy vegetables are the best and will help your body drop weight faster than you may think. Scientists are still uncertain as to why green leafy vegetables promote rapid weight loss, but try consuming at least 3 servings (5 cups) a week and see what it does for you.

Green Leafy Vegetables Include:

Spinach – This leafy green is packed with iron, calcium, and vitamin K. Spinach is typically available year round, in organic and conventional bags. It can be expensive but during the summer it is usually the cheapest.

Kale – A dark fibrous leafy green that has a slightly bitter taste. Kale is full of beta carotene, vitamin k, vitamin c, lutein, calcium, and sulforaphane which is shown to have anti-cancer benefits to the body. Kale takes some time to cook, but you can boil, steam, microwave, and stirfry this vegetable. It is also excellent in green smoothies.

Kohlrabi – This plant is related to cabbage but has a sweeter and milder taste than other bitter greens. It looks funny and may be hard to find, but also contains tons of potent nutrients. It is also hardy and can grow in any condition, making it great for those that don't live near farming communities.

Cabbage – Green and somewhat bitter, cabbage is an excellent detoxifying vegetable. Cabbage in soups and stews will help you flush excess salts and toxins from the body while providing cancer fighting antioxidants.

Romaine – This green leafy vegetable is light in flavor and the healthier cousin of lettuce. Use romaine for your salads if you are a beginner, or blend it into a green smoothie. Romaine has chlorophyll properties to help prevent colon and liver cancers.

Baby Romaine – This is the young version of romaine lettuce. It is more tender and soft.

Broccolini – This unique vegetable is often thought of as young broccoli, but that would be a misconception. This tender veggie is long and has small florets at the tops of long stalks. It is grown in California and Arizona, and available year round. Broccolini is high in folate, Vitamin c, calcium and iron.

Brussels Sprouts – These little vegetables are related to wild cabbage but firm, round, and small. Most people cringe at the thought of trying Brussels sprouts, but they are truly some of the healthiest things you can eat, and extremely cheap. These contain the same sulforaphane compound that has potent anticancer properties. Another interesting thing is that Brussels sprouts contain indole-3-carbinol, which is a chemical that helps your body repair damaged DNA from free radicals. It also blocks cancer growth.

Bok Choy – This Chinese green contains high vitamin a and vitamin c per 4 ounce serving. It must be cooked very well to prevent toxicity problems.

Chard – This colorful vegetable is a root and related to the beet root. It is also known as Swiss chard. It is extremely prone to bruising and perishing, so it is best to eat it the same day you buy it. Chard is slightly bitter but when cooked it has a delicate taste and is less noticeable than spinach. This green is extremely high in vitamins A, K, and C. It also has a lot of fiber and even protein.

Mustard – These greens are spicy and bitter and commonly used in Southern, Asian and Indian cuisines. It contains a number of vitamins as well, especially iron and zinc.

Rutabaga – These root vegetables are an excellent choice for sweet but healthy dishes. They are best mashed like potatoes with light milk and a tiny bit of butter.

Collards – These greens are grown around the world, but they are particularly popular in the Southern United States. These greens are classified with Kale but taste a bit different. They are very low in calories like all greens, and provide a rich flavor to any dish. They are packed with vitamin c, fiber, and anti-cancer properties.

Chicory Vegetables – This group of vegetables consists of greens like Endive. It is a semi-uncommon produce in the

United States but can be eaten raw or in salads. It is especially high in fiber and folate, Vitamins A and K.

There are many more to choose from, but the above leafy greens are the most common and easy to find. They are even extremely affordable, particularly Kale. The USDA recommends at least 3 cups a week of dark leafy greens, which is easy to do once you get in the habit of it. In fact, most restaurant and fast food salads contain that many cups in just one salad as long as it is not plain lettuce. To make prepared salads a healthier option for you, skip cheese, rich dressings, fried chicken, and croutons. Use vinaigrette instead or a light dressing, and choose grilled chicken, tofu, or raw nuts for protein.

Why choose green leafy vegetables? For one, they are some of the most powerful nutrition sources on the planet. Leafy greens are packed with phytonutrients, iron, potassium, calcium, and protein. Since they are low in calories, with spinach only having 7 calories per cup, the nutritional amounts in each serving of greens are astounding.

Greens protect the body from free radicals, cancer, age related conditions, disease, and sickness. The best part is that they will help you shed weight due to high fiber and water content. Once you start consuming leafy greens on a daily or at least weekly basis, your body will thank you.

Other non-starchy vegetables include:

Amaranth – This is an interesting vegetable, as it is usually seen as a weed. But amaranth makes a great cereal grain, leafy vegetable, and an herb as well. Amaranth is full of vitamin A, C, folate, thiamine, niacin, riboflavin, calcium, and zinc. It is best to cook the grain or eat it as part of a cereal blend. This super food is an ancient grain, and full of enzymes and important amino acids for optimal health.

Artichoke – They are complicated to cook but delicious and worth the work to eat them. Artichokes require you to remove all of the excess leaves and cutting away parts of the stem. This removes thorns and other inedible parts of the plant. Boiling or steaming until tender results in the best flavor.

Artichoke hearts – These are the core of the artichoke and are edible once everything else is removed. The hearts are rich in fiber and chlorophyll, which is partially destroyed during cooking. To eat artichoke hearts it is best to make dips with them. They are also great on sandwiches and paired with spinach.

Asparagus – This is technically a spring veggie but can be found almost year round. Asparagus is very low in calories, and has B6, calcium, magnesium, and zinc. It is also low in carbohydrates and packed with protein and other sources of vitamins, minerals, and metals that the body needs. It even contains chromium which is shown to help blood sugar stay balanced and reduce weight. If you want to shed pounds faster, eat your asparagus.

Beans – Green beans that is. These are low in carbohydrates but packed full of fiber and other vitamins. Green beans are cheap, a fall food, and excellent paired with mostly any meal. The best part is that most people already enjoy green beans. If you rely on canned ones, try buying fresh green beans and cooking them from scratch. You will not want to go back to canned beans again.

Bean sprouts – Sprouts are created by soaking germinating beans in water for a period of time. The sprouting allows the new plant to emerge, which can then be eaten on salads and sandwiches. Bean sprouts are safe to eat raw or cooked, but eating them raw carries some risk. They may contribute to bacterial infections in the colon, or in worst cases in systemic bacterial diseases. Their high enzymes and nutritious benefits make them the ideal food for those trying to lose weight within moderation in their raw state.

Beets – These dark purple and red colored roots are an excellent addition to your diet if you can learn to like them. They can cure constipation, boost digestive ability, and even protect your skin and body against oxidation and free radicals.

Broccoli – This winter veggie is common and well loved by many. Packed with folate and calcium, broccoli is the perfect thing to throw in soups and meals to add vitamins to your diet. It is also very affordable when it is in season.

Carrots – Yet another favorite root vegetable, carrots are high in beta carotene and low in calories. These sweet crunchy roots make great snacks or cooked in stews and soups. They can be honeyed, boiled or steamed. Carrots pair well with other vegetables as well.

Cauliflower – These veggie looks like white broccoli and seems useless to many, but actually has dozens of health benefits. It is cheap, low in fat and very high in fiber and water, and has a high nutritional density cup per cup. It is packed with sulforaphane, glucoinolates, cartenoids, and indole-3-carbinol. These powerful compounds are a super defense for your body. Instead of potatoes, you can mash cauliflower to create something low-carb that tastes very similar.

Celery – A very low calorie food, celery has been thought to contain negative calories. This means it takes more energy for your body to digest it than it provides. It is an excellent food for weight loss and has extremely high fiber content.

Chayote – This is a bland pear vegetable that has minimal flavor unless it is cooked. It is full of amino acids, Vitamin C and fiber.

Cucumber – They are often seen as a vegetable but are technically a fruit. They are sweet but low in carbohydrates and calories. They contain trace minerals and vitamins and make an excellent topper for a sandwich or salad. Cucumber spears are great as a snack.

Eggplant – This interesting fruit is classified as a berry, and is fleshy and often used as a meat replacement. It tastes similar to bell peppers and other berry "pepper" plants, but it is related to tomatoes and tobacco. Eggplant is effective at lowering high cholesterol. If you suffer from cholesterol problems, then consume eggplant a few times per week to help lower your cholesterol. It is also full of folic acid and potassium. You can make a healthy pizza by using eggplant, or grilling slabs of the fruit and making a sandwich.

Green onions or scallions – These are excellent diced and added to foods for a little extra flavor. Green onions also have antioxidant properties.

Jicama – This root vegetable is not everyone's cup of tea, but it is very common in the Southwest. Made primarily of water it is low in everything but fiber. It has a high concentration of a unique pre-biotic as well, making it a great snack to aid in digestion.

Leeks – The stalk and bulb of the leek are the edible portions that contain the most nutrients and flavor. They are often added to soups and foods and rarely eaten alone. Use leeks to add flavor to Asian style dishes and soups, without the bitter taste of a green onion.

Mushrooms – There are dozens of types of mushrooms and each one has its own beneficial properties. White button mushrooms are common and very cheap, and packed with anti-aging nutrients. Portobello mushroom caps are excellent baked or grilled for sandwiches or alone. Stuffing mushrooms is a great way to have a meat free meal packed with flavor. Mushrooms are great for the skin and are shown to prevent wrinkles.

Okra – It tastes good as a steamed vegetable or mixed with other foods, but has few notable nutritional benefits. Since it is a natural food though, it should be consumed if you enjoy it!

Onions – They are often seen as an empty root that makes you cry, but onions actually possess anti-cancerous benefits.

Daikon – A huge serving of this root contains only 6 calories but has at least 34% of the recommended amount of Vitamin C that you need, per 100 gram serving. The storage life is not long for Daikon and it should be eaten as soon as possible. It is excellent in stews.

Pea pods – What isn't there to enjoy about pea pods? They are packed with iron and fiber and make salads crunchy and delicious. The whole pea pod is edible raw or cooked, but may taste best slightly steamed.

Peppers – All peppers, including bell peppers and jalapeno, habanero, and sweet peppers, contain potent anti-oxidant properties, are low in calories, and help the body fight cancer. They are readily available and taste great added to mostly any meal.

Radishes – These small roots are often used in salad mixes but taste a little bitter. They are an excellent source of ascorbic acid, folates, potassium, b6 vitamins, magnesium, and even calcium. They are low in calories but made primarily of carbohydrates.

Sauerkraut – This is a fermented cabbage but is full of lactic acid bacteria and has a long shelf life. Despite how gross that sounds, Sauerkraut is actually very nutritious and provides vitamin C and other bacteria that is beneficial to the body. Sauerkraut isn't for everyone, but does make an excellent cancer fighting stored food.

Sugar snap peas – These winter veggies are served whole and taste best that way, too. They are great steamed and provide significant fiber.

Summer squash – All squash plants are great for your health since they contain antioxidants and fiber, without many carbohydrates.

Tomato – This fruit is often considered a veggie, but is a huge source of lycopene, which is great for men and women. It fights prostate cancer and improves the skin. Look for deep red tomatoes and choose on the vine when available.

Zucchini – This green squash grows almost anywhere and is very easy to cultivate, even for novice gardeners. Zucchini is extremely low in calories, high in water content and protein, and packed with vitamins. It makes a great side dish steamed or grilled, and can even be shredded to form patties.

A few of the above non-starchy vegetables should be consumed each day, except for breakfast. Choose what you like the most and rotate on a weekly basis. One week select 5 different non-starchy vegetables that you enjoy. Then on week two, change things up a bit. This ensures you get diversity in your diet. Becoming bored with vegetables is a dieter's worst enemy. Making them into snacks is also a great way to get your vegetable servings in. Non-starchy veggies are low in carbohydrates but high in important nutrients that your body relies on for weight loss, brain health, and other bodily functions.

To reach the ideal amount, women should consume two and a half cups of vegetables per day, and men should have three cups. It is acceptable to consume up to six cups of vegetables each day if you are able to do so. However, even the minimum will help aid in weight loss and a complete healthy lifestyle change.

Fruits

Fruits are something most people tend to enjoy. They are sweet, nutritious, and make you feel like you are enjoying a nice treat without overindulging in junk food. Fruits also provide water, nutrients, fiber, and antioxidants that defend against aging.

Fruits To Consume:

Apples - These cheap fruits are available year round and come in a dozen of types from classic Red Delicious to sweet Pink Ladies and Fiji apples. They are loaded with fiber, and often come with the classic phrase "an apple a day keeps the doctor away." It turns out this phrase is relatively true.

Apricots - While they are most common in spring, dried varieties can be found year round. Apricots are soft and slightly sour with a tinge of sweetness. Apricots are surprisingly nutritional powerhouses, as they contain large amounts of a diverse range of carotenoids. These antioxidants are special because they may help fight against heart disease and reduce cholesterol. Not only that, but apricots are great for hydration and regular bowel movements. Keeping unsweetened dried apricots around is a great way to keep your body regular.

Bananas - Packed with potassium, a banana makes a great pre-workout snack. Many people suggest eating only half a banana due to the carbohydrates. In reality, a whole banana is much better for you than any other processed snack. The average banana only contains 13 carbohydrates.

Raspberries - These tart, brightly colored berries are easy to eat, low in calories, and full of polyphenol antioxidants and anthocyanins. These compounds protect the body against disease and nourish the skin from the inside out. They are high in fiber as well and known as an anti aging powerhouse.

Strawberries - The classic strawberry is more like a delicious dessert than a nutritious food. But aside from what our taste buds think, strawberries are full of fiber and other minerals such as calcium and strong antioxidants that come from their red coloring.

Blueberries - These berries are packed with weight loss and anti-disease properties. They are full of anthocyanins, the antioxidant pigment that many berries contain. They can reduce inflammation in the body when enough are consumed, and taste great in smoothies, on cakes and tarts, and as part of your everyday cereal. Blueberries are perfect dried as well.

Cherries – This is yet another red pigmented berry full of skin and body-benefiting nutrients. These reduce inflammation and pain when consumed frequently. Cherries aid in weight loss, cholesterol reduction, and triglyceride reduction.

Grapefruit - This fruit is often used as a weight loss tool, because it is said to boost metabolism. Grapefruits are very energizing and provide a lot of fiber. Half of a grapefruit a day can be beneficial for losing weight.

Grapes - All types of grapes, which are used to make wine, are a great way to get powerful antioxidants on the cheap. Portable, small, and easy to eat, grapes are high in water content and low in calories. Their sweet or sour taste makes them almost like nature's candy.

Kiwi - These green fuzzy fruits are actually a winter fruit. They contain high levels of water as well as potassium.

Mangoes - A tropical favorite, mangoes are full of fiber, Vitamin c, Vitamin a, and carotenoids. Higher in calories than many fruits, mangoes still provide excellent nutritional benefit.

Cantaloupe - These melons have polyphenols and provide immune system strength and cardiovascular health. Eating cantaloupe will help you power through your workouts and lose weight faster. Eat as much as you would like, because melons are superior in nutrition.

Honeydew - These melons have all of the same benefits as cantaloupe but a slightly sweeter taste. Some people prefer to eat cantaloupe and honeydew together.

Watermelon - The bright pink and red colors of watermelon, and the high water content, make it a summer-time favorite. Watermelon is an excellent hydrator, extremely low in calories, and provides sustainable energy to the body. It is also said to boost weight loss.

Oranges - Packed with Vitamin C, oranges are easy to find and cheap to buy. They are available year round and have many different types that have slightly different tastes.

Peaches – Sweet, and available in summer to fall, peaches are perfect for sautéing and topping on sorbets or making fruit mixes and pies from. Packed with carotenoids and fiber, peaches are a delicious way to get your servings of fruit in.

Pears - These are a winter fruit that are similar to an apple but softer and sweeter to most. They pack 6 grams of fiber per fruit, making them excellent for regularity.

Papaya - The phytochemicals in papaya are great for the skin and body. They provide plenty of energy and hydration as well.

Pineapple - These sweet fruits are high in glycemic characteristics, but great topped on burgers and grilled.

Pineapple also contains carotenoids and is excellent for fiber content.

Plums - Dark plums are a great source of sweet juicy flesh and potent antioxidants. They are also known to have tons of fiber that promotes regularity.

Prunes - Dried plums are another source of high fiber and vitamin content. Buy these without sugar added.

Raisins - Dried grapes are a great way to add fiber to your oatmeal, cereal, breads, muffins, and treats.

While fruit juices and fruit cocktails do constitute as a serving of fruit, for the purpose of weight loss you should avoid these. If you must drink fruit juice, make sure it is 100% juice not from concentrate and contains no added sugars.

Women and men can enjoy two cups of fruits per day for optimum health and balance. Up to five cups of low-glycemic fruits are allowed as long as they fit within the calorie budget.

Choose organic versions of the dirty dozen if possible. This includes berries, mango, apples, and grapes. Not everyone has easy access to organic food, but it is important to choose them when you can.

Whole Grains
Avoiding processed refined grains is another step in the right direction to formulating a balanced diet. Whole grains are not processed or are processed minimally. When you consume whole grains you will be adding significant amounts of fiber, protein, and nutrients to your diet. Grains are necessary for

lower cholesterol and helping your digestive system stay regular.

A whole grain is considered the entire grain kernel – the bran, germ, and endosperm. Breads and pastas often do not contain the whole grain. There are processed options that do tout whole grain, and you should look for those. It is essential to avoid anything white and refined, enriched, or stone ground. These keywords should be red flags when shopping for healthy groceries.

There is a whole grain out there for everyone. Whole wheat flour, spelt, amaranth, bulgur, oatmeal, whole cornmeal, and brown rice are the basics. You can also incorporate quinoa and other "exotic" whole grains for optimum health.

If you are trying to make a healthy diet change for weight loss, but have gluten intolerance, there are plenty of grains out there without gluten. Supermarkets are stocking more gluten-free products as well, so that you can still eat whole grains without the irritable bowel problems.

You do not need enriched grains if they are true whole grains. Grains will retain their nutrients and minerals without having them added back in.

At least 40 grams of whole grains are recommended per day. There are many cereals out there that make up a number of those grams, and include at least 10 grams of fiber and protein as well. Choosing the right servings of grains is based on your dietary needs. If you are vegetarian or vegan you will be eating more of them. Be sure to balance the calories and carbohydrates into your diet, and that is all that matters when it comes to determining serving amounts. If this is difficult for you, then go for about four ounces of whole grains per day.

Types Of Grains:

Quinoa – This is a grain that isn't really a grain, but for dietary purposes it is treated as such. Quinoa is a seed-like food that has a grassy taste if not cooked properly. However, after proper soaking and preparation it has a very light flavor that goes well in a number of dishes. Quinoa is very high in protein, and has much more than wheat and rice. This is fantastic for those that are trying to eat less meat. Quinoa also contains a complete protein, which means it has everything people need to build muscle. Complete plant proteins are rare.

Amaranth – This was also listed as a vegetable, but amaranth is used in cereals quite commonly. It is a good source of Vitamin A, C, and folate, and contains other vitamins as well. It is best to eat amaranth with oats, wheat germ, and other grains because they form a complete protein together.

Wheat – Classic, delicious, and widely used in food, wheat is an affordable choice for bread and cooking needs in their wholegrain form.

Spelt – This grain is considered an ancient grain and is very similar to wheat. However the health benefits are a bit different. It is high in protein and fiber. It is alright for baking sometimes but not all of the time, depending on what you cook. Spelt makes great bread products, but can over-thicken soups and stews.

Brown Rice – When making a lifestyle change every source says to switch to brown rice instead of white rice. This is because brown rice still retains the germ and natural grain. It is chewy and contains much more fiber than fluffy white rice. Brown rice has a shorter shelf life so you should eat it relatively soon after buying it if possible.

Black Rice – Most people have never seen black rice, let alone consumed it. This rice is usually hidden on health food store shelves in smaller bags. It usually isn't much more expensive either. Black rice is packed with iron and fiber, and tastes about the same as brown rice. The difference is the iron content and very high anthocyanin levels. If you want to switch things up, reach for black rice instead of brown.

Barley – This diverse grain is used in a number of things from beer to animal food. Barley itself is soft and delicate and has the ability to regulate glucose levels. Barley is excellent in soups, so make a point to eat it frequently if you are concerned about glucose levels.

Bulgur – This grain is a cereal type food that is excellent to eat hot for breakfast. It is high in protein, fiber, has a relatively low glycemic index. One full cup of dry bulgur contains 25 grams of fiber. Most people would only eat a half cup or less, but even when you break the numbers down it is a significant amount of fiber.

Corn – Most people assume corn to be a vegetable. Corn is in fact a grain, and eating it whole on the cob is the best way. Roasted corn with spices makes a great snack or side dish. Skip the butter and creamy sauce for a delicious whole grain choice.

Durum – This wheat is not your typical wheat. It is higher in protein than many wheat species and extremely hard compared to normal wheat. It is low in gluten as well. This wheat is used to make bread but it isn't highly recommended. This wheat is great for pasta and macaroni.

Fonio – You may have never heard of this grain, because it is very small and grown in Africa. It is related to millet. It is extremely nutritious, cheap, and grows very fast. You can harvest fonio within 2 months and it grows very well in arid areas. If you find fonio, prepare it as a hot cereal.

Kamut – This is a large wheat grain that is rich in taste and has a nutty flavor. Kamut has about 14 grams of protein per 3.5 ounces, which is significant for a grain. It is high-energy and has complex carbohydrates that other grains do not. When it is processed into flour or ground, it doesn't lose as much nutrition as other grains. Kamut is a great side dish for preparing healthy ethnic meals, or if you prefer to grind your own flour it, makes great healthy breads.

Millet – This major food source is a choice amongst those that live in arid and semi-arid climates, particularly India. For that reason, millet is great for homemade Indian cuisine. Millet is an excellent choice for those that suffer from celiac disease, as it does not contain gluten. It has less protein than many types of wheat but is high in B Vitamins.

Oats – These are well known grains that fill you with fiber and lower bad cholesterol. Many packages of oats also say that it will reduce your risk of heart disease. Oats are digested slowly since their fiber content is soluble and helps you feel full for hours after eating a bowl of oats. Oat bran is also a great way to add extra soluble fiber to your diet. Oats are cheap, delicious, and go great with fruits and other sweet spices such as cinnamon and nutmeg.

Rye – This grain is commonly used in rye bread and offers a rich flavor compared to regular wheat bread. It also has a high amount of soluble fiber and is lower in gluten.

Teff – This grain is very expensive in the United States because it is native to Ethiopia. Teff is extremely high in fiber and iron, as well as protein and calcium. The most common way it is used is by making teff tortillas or teff wraps. These healthy alternatives to flour tortillas provide a rich and nutritious wrap for vegetables and whatever fillings you enjoy.

Triticale – This wheat and rye hybrid grain is commonly used in hot cereal blends. It is nutritious and rich and makes a great add-in for 10 grain cereals or multigrain foods.

Buckwheat – This is not a true grass or wheat, but is still considered a grain. Buckwheat is made into flours and can be used for a number of baking purposes. It is also used in pasta.

Chia – These tiny seeds are best known by their 1990s craze of "Chia Pets." When planted they sprout green grass. When consumed as a seed, chia is packed with omega-3 fatty acids, fiber, and numerous health benefits. Adding chia to smoothies and baked goods or even juices and pudding will provide you with an energizing health boost.

Dairy and Dairy Substitutes
Dairy products provide calcium, Vitamin D, protein, and make a great energizer for those trying to lose weight. Most people consume too much high fat dairy, such as full fat milk, cheeses, ice cream, and other dairy products. Instead of full fat varieties, choose low fat or skim dairy, no-sugar-added

yogurts, and avoid ice cream. Low-fat frozen yogurt is a better choice.

Adults should have three cups of low-fat dairy products per day. This will provide the right amount of protein and calcium to keep your muscles fueled. If you have a dairy allergy or intolerance, there are plenty of fortified replacements on the market. Soy milk, almond milk, coconut milk, hemp milk, and oat milk are all available. There are even nut cheeses and ice creams too. All of the above-mentioned have the same amount of calcium and nutrients as conventional dairy, but no cholesterol and minimal saturated fats. Any of these substitutes are perfectly acceptable and will still fuel your body with what it needs to be strong and healthy. Additionally, they taste great.

Almond Milk – Made from blended and separated almonds, this milk is creamy and rich and easily comparable to cows' milk. It has Vitamin D and calcium, and is very low in calories. This milk makes a great choice for those trying to watch fat and calorie intake, as 1 cup only has 35 to 40 calories. Adding it to cereal or cooked foods can further reduce calorie intake.

Soy Milk – Popular and the most common milk replacement, soy milk is considered a whole food. Purchase the organic unsweetened kind for the best health benefits. It is packed with soy protein, Vitamin D, calcium, B Vitamins, iron, and other nutrients that cows' milk provides. It is also low in calories.

Hemp Milk – This milk is made from hulled hemp seeds. It is very rich and grassy and provides a complete protein. This unique flavor of milk isn't for everyone but it is a very powerful super-food with numerous health benefits.

Coconut Milk – While coconut milk is high in saturated fat, it comes from medium-chain fatty acids and not long-chain fatty acids. Medium chains are healthy and provide your body with the "good fat" that it needs. Coconut milk is low in calories but packed with unique nutrients you won't find in other types of milk. There are also different flavors of coconut milk to try. Adding it to cereals and oatmeal makes an excellent light treat.

Oat Milk – Made from oat bran, oat milk is creamy and rich in nutrients. You may need fortified versions to get the proper nutrients if you drink it frequently.

Rice Milk – Similar to the Mexican treat Horchata, rice milk is fortified to have all of the nutrients you need such as calcium and iron. It has moderate caloric values. However, rice milk has a delicious flavor that many people prefer over other alternatives.

Rice Cheeses – These cheeses are made with rice milk instead of cows' milk. They taste very similar to "normal" cheese but do not contain lactose. They are ideal for those with allergies. Rice cheese also comes in flavors such as American slices, Pepper Jack, Cheddar, and Mozzarella.

Almond and Nut Cheeses – These cheeses are made with the fat of nuts, commonly almond and cashew. They are rich and often extremely close to cow cheese. They are a specialty cheese and therefore more expensive than conventional cow or goat cheeses. The taste is undeniable however.

Other Vegan Cheeses – Expert food crafting technology has made it possible for tons of vegan cheeses to be produced.

They are often just as gooey and tasty as cow cheese, but are safe for those with allergies to soy, lactose, and nuts.

Lean Proteins

Proteins consist of meat products such as fish, lamb, pork, beef, chicken, and turkey. Additionally tofu, beans, and legumes also count as a protein. When making protein choices for weight loss, always choose small grilled lean portions. Purchasing extra lean meat is the most beneficial thing for your body, and it helps to weigh out your portions.

Women only need about 4-5 ounces of lean meat per day, while men need about 6 ounces. Beef is not included in this, as the recommended amount of beef per WEEK is a 5 ounce serving. Avoiding red meat is a great way to help with weight loss while consuming higher quality proteins.

Vegetarians and vegans can choose tofu, legumes, beans, and tempeh for their protein needs. While all other food products contain protein, these foods contain the most that your body needs. It's relatively easy and cheap to have 5 ounces or less of these proteins per day, and they are already naturally low in fat!

Fats and Oils

Everyone can benefit from healthy fats, and they should be incorporated into your diet. Healthy fats include avocado, nuts, and high quality olive oil. Since they do contain omega-3 fatty acids, it is important to not overdo them on any given day. Limit your healthy fats to 1.5 ounces of nuts per day. Oils should be kept to a tablespoon or less per day.

Coconut Oil – When purchasing coconut oil, look for organic extra virgin. This means it is unrefined and is still retaining all of the complex nutrients. Coconut oil is great for high heat cooking and adds a light deliciously sweet flavor to meals. It is also packed with omega-3. You can top popcorn with coconut oil as well.

Walnut Oil – This type of oil is expensive but has a rich nutty taste, and is also packed with beneficial omega-3 fatty acids.

Canola Oil – Choose organic oil if possible. Conventional canola oil is produced with GMO plants and is not as high quality as an organic version. Also look for high heat canola oil for the best results.

Olive Oil – Great for cold meals or as a dip or sauce. Do not use olive oil to cook if you can prevent it. Heating olive oil destroys the health properties and makes it worse for you than other types of oils.

Sesame Oil – This is ideal for cooking Asian inspired dishes and preparing a homemade Asian type dressing for salads.

Cooking oils can add flavor and pizzazz to boring "health food" so use them, but be sure to use them sparingly to ensure that you don't go overboard with calories and fat.

2.1 - The Importance of Nutrition

Now that we have covered the basics of a balanced diet, we can start to discuss the importance of proper nutrition for weight loss. This can become confusing for those new to dieting, but it is all fairly simple to follow once you know why it is necessary.

The average diet in America is composed of fast food, processed foods, and empty calories. Even home cooked meals tend to be partially processed. Most people buy canned corn instead of fresh. Fewer people purchase fresh green beans, and instead go for canned ones. This accumulates a significant amount of sodium into your diet that causes high blood pressure and other potential health risks. Processed foods also lose many of their nutrients. This is why if you look at the nutrition label on apple juice, it seems like it has nothing beneficial compared to a fresh apple.

What foods are "good" and which foods are "bad", though? Magazines, diet books, the Internet, and countless other sources will give you conflicting information. One source will say to eat beef; another will say avoid red meat at all costs. One source will encourage processed foods, while another says avoid all of them.

The things every person should look out for include:

- Refined grains. Think of white bread, white flour, and white pasta. These are usually lacking all of the great vitamins and minerals that whole grains have. They leave you feeling hungry after eating and do not provide lasting energy.

- Refined sugars. Think of candy bars, ice cream, boxed cereals that are not specifically low in sugar/no sugar, dairy products with added sugar, white sugar, doughnuts, and all other sweet treats.

- High fat meats. These are high in saturated and trans fats, which lead to heart disease, diabetes, and high cholesterol. It is shocking for people to hear that high fat diets do lead to diabetes.

- Organ meats. These are also high in fat and bad for your heart and liver.

- Aged meats such as sausages, pepperoni, and other non-lean high fat deli meats. These contain high levels of chemicals used to process these foods into sausages and pepperoni. Aged meats are notoriously bad for your heart and liver.

- High sodium frozen foods. Sodium aids in bloating and can lead to hypertension. If you want to lose weight consistently, lower your sodium intake.

- High sodium canned foods. See the above for reasons on why you should avoid this.

- High fructose corn syrup is known to cause addiction to sugars and treats, as well as a dramatically increased the chance of developing type-2 diabetes. Even cane sugar is a better choice over high fructose corn syrup. Eliminate this from your diet, even if you have difficulty removing other things.

The above lists the primary things to watch out for in order to lose weight and be a healthy individual. Even seemingly healthy processed foods can take a toll on your health, and your weight loss. For example, many "healthy" frozen meals contain over 800mg of sodium per meal. Most are made with inferior ingredients, very little fresh food, and are high in refined carbohydrates. While the basic nutritional guidelines on the packages sound decent, they lack the ability to nurture your body for a lengthy period of time. Not only that, but most packaged meals marketed to dieters are less than 350 calories. This is a very small amount for lunch or dinner, especially for someone that is exercising.

Choosing the right foods during grocery shopping and at meal times can be a hassle and a confusing process. The important thing to remember is circle the perimeter of the store first. Inner isles typically contain processed foods, junk food, and otherwise unhealthy products. The perimeter is where you find dairy, proteins, fruits, veggies, and bulk grains.

When grocery shopping look for food that meets this criteria:

- Has at least one gram of fiber per serving. The more fiber, the better.

- Does not have sugar listed as one of the first few ingredients.

- Contains whole grains if the product is a grain based food.

- Soy should be organic whenever possible.

- If frozen or processed, look for less than 700mg of sodium per package.

- Avoid sugary drinks and juices.

- Stick with a cart full of produce, lean meat, grains, dairy, and legumes.

How Much and When to Eat
The fine details of how much and when to eat are equally as important as what you are eating. There are tons of

guidelines for when and how to eat your food, but the main thing to remember is that less is more. Smaller portion sizes are always going to be a safe bet for your diet.

Women should aim to consume about 1,200 to 1,500 calories per day. The exact amount depends on your exercise intensity. If you exercise for more than an hour at a high intensity, your body needs more calories. Additionally, heavier people will need more food.

Men should aim for 1,400-1,800 calories per day. Most men are given 1,800 calories as their guidelines, but it should be based on how you feel.

Never rely on just your calorie intake. You must factor in fat, protein, and carbohydrates as well. You can consume 1,200 calories with 70 grams of protein and 30 grams of fiber and feel completely full. On the other hand, eating 1,200 calories with only 30 grams of protein and almost no fiber, will leave you starving. Keep your meals balanced and you will never be hungry while trying to lose weight.

To determine a good amount of calories for your body, do a simple BMR calculation. Your BMR is your basal metabolic rate, in other words, what you burn while you are resting. The formula is:

Women: BMR = 655 + (4.35 x weight in pounds) + (4.7 x height in inches) - (4.7 x age in years)
Men: BMR = 66 + (6.23 x weight in pounds) + (12.7 x height in inches) - (6.8 x age in year)

This amount will help you gauge what you should be consuming for weight loss. Your BMR decreases the older you get, but it increases with increased exercise and activity. If your BMR is 2,000 you should aim for about 1,500 calories consumed, and an additional 250 calories burned for optimal weight loss. Your BMR may be slightly different from your true BMR number, so take it with a grain of salt. Either way, eating significantly under will help you lose weight if you are consistent.

Another important thing is to force your body into the habit of eating three core meals per day, breakfast, lunch, and dinner. Eat breakfast foods when you first wake up, then lunch four hours later, then dinner four hours after that. In between snack on fruits and veggies or other low-calorie snacks that are less than 150 calories per serving. Frequent consumption of food will keep you full. If you let yourself go too long without eating to "save calories" you are going to be cranky and likely to overeat on sugary junk food.

Throughout the day you should aim to divide your weight in half and drink that much in ounces. For example, if you weigh 200 pounds, you should consume 100 ounces of water. This is the base number. If you exercise, you should add 20 ounces. If you live in an arid climate, add 20 more ounces. Your body needs more water than previously thought, and the minimum of 64 ounces isn't enough anymore. If you find it difficult to drink that much water, you can supplement with unsweetened teas.

Choosing Good Foods While Eating Out
Despite your efforts to lose weight and be healthy, you will be faced with situations where you will need to eat out at a restaurant or fast food establishment. More places are working to provide people with healthier options while dining

out. Remember that portion sizes are important and restaurants often have huge portions. A McDonald's Big Mac Value Meal can pack on over 1,000 calories if you choose a medium size. This doesn't even include a sugary soda. Knowing how to navigate your way around a menu will allow you to enjoy time out with friends and family without making a sacrifice.

This might sound shocking, but it is highly recommended that you avoid the typical restaurant salad. The Chili's Boneless Buffalo Chicken salad for example, sits at over 1,000 calories, 77 grams of fat, and double the recommended sodium intake. One of the biggest mistakes dieters make while dining out is ordering a salad like this, and thinking that it is healthy.

Instead of that type of salad, order a lean grilled piece of chicken, a side of steamed veggies, and a small side salad. You can also look at the healthy sections restaurants have designated for people trying to eat healthier while dining out.

Always avoid anything creamy, sautéed, savory, buttery, and crispy. Essentially any menu item ending with a "y" will likely be bad for you. Instead aim for grilled, steamed, light, and seasoned. When you are ordering sandwiches or burgers skip dressings and cheese toppings. If you must have dressings then order it on the side to apply an appropriate amount. These pack on useless calories that add to weight gain or negate your hard work for shedding pounds.

Most restaurants will allow you to order a heaping side of steamed plain veggies, so go with that option when possible. If there are doubts on how the vegetables are prepared, ask your server. You can request light butter or oil, or none at all.

It is perfectly acceptable to ask your server for special accommodations.

How Good Food Benefits Your Body Inside And Out
The building blocks of a strong healthy body, starts with a healthy diet. Vitamins, minerals, protein, and even fats and sugars, all help your body stay in tip-top shape, fight aging, disease, and illness. When your body starts to lack an important vital nutrient, you start to feel the symptoms of vitamin deficiency. It can take quite awhile to get to that point, but millions of people in the United States alone are affected by malnutrition. Even overweight and obese people can be malnourished, which leads to dizziness, constant fatigue, frequent sickness, dramatic weight changes, slowed metabolism, and much more.

Once you make a lifestyle change and fill your body with nutrients, you will alleviate the majority of the problems you experience with your health. Diabetes can be reduced dramatically by following a moderate carbohydrate diet full of vegetables and lean protein. Headaches and fatigue can be erased by eating leafy greens and getting a balanced meal 3 times per day. Memory function is strengthened by eating omega-3 fatty acids. You can find those in walnuts, flaxseeds, fish, pumpkin seeds, and countless other foods.

Internally your body will fight off disease, viruses, and bacterial infections. Externally you will look radiant, your skin will become resilient, and you will age at a slower rate than those consuming a diet of fast food and processed dinners.

One of the scariest effects of a diet high in refined sugar is the rate at which sugar increases wrinkles. Sugar has been shown to breakdown collagen and cause loss of elasticity in the skin. This promotes rapid aging. Instead of sugar, eat fruits that are packed with beneficial antioxidants. Grapes, particularly dark red or black ones, are shown to promote healthy wrinkle-free skin.

The important thing to know is that good foods will heal you from the inside to the outside. From your bones to your organs, this miraculous process takes place. It may not be noticeable immediately, but in 10 years you will not regret treating your body to healthy fulfilling foods.

Eating healthy foods to lose weight will:

- Reduce your risk of type-2 diabetes.

- Reduce your risk of heart disease.

- Reduce your risk of cancer.

- Improve your quality of life.

- Lengthen your potential life span.

- Reverse the problems caused by type-2 diabetes if you are already diabetic.

- Fight the signs of aging including superficial skin problems, joint pain, and the general "slow down" that happens as you age.

- Berries are shown to defend against Alzheimer's, so consume them frequently to fuel your brain and keep your memory strong.

2.2 - Good Foods

Why You Should Be Limiting Sugars and Carbohydrates

This isn't a low-carb diet spiel. In fact, low-carb diets are more harmful than beneficial. However, anyone trying to lose weight can benefit from limiting sugars and carbohydrates in their daily diet. Sugars, particularly refined ones, spike glucose levels and lead to a crash. When you eat a candy bar your sugar level goes high to give your body energy. When that energy is not used, your body "crashes" and feels fatigued and exhausted. Sugar rush is an accurate term to describe what happens. On the other hand, eating a food bar with low-glycemic properties, less carbohydrates, and high protein, can prevent these crashes.

While some people argue that there is no such thing as good carbs and bad carbs, this is largely a myth that diet book writers promote. Good carbohydrates are the low-glycemic variety. They are packed with fiber, protein, and other nutrients. Bad carbohydrates are the kind found in candy, sugar, ice cream, refined breads, white pasta, and other junk food. These products contain little to no fiber or protein, minimal nutrients, and offer your body no health benefits.

The Diabetic Association suggests that eating 180 carbohydrates per day is an effective amount to shed at least 2 pounds per week and reverse the problems that diabetes can bring to the surface. When most of those carbohydrates are low-glycemic and filled with fiber, you will feel full longer and have stabilized energy throughout the day. Even if you are not diabetic, it can be beneficial to follow some of their guidelines for prevention and weight loss.

If you do not believe this information, try following your calorie guidelines and eating whatever you want for one day. Don't think about carbohydrates and sugar, but stick with your calorie range. Notice how you feel fatigued, cranky, and constantly hungry. Now fill your meals with whole grains, carbohydrates from fruit, and low-glycemic foods. You will stay full for longer, have steady energy, and sleep better at night.

Low-Glycemic Sugars

If you can't have conventional sugars, then what can you have? The answer is low-glycemic sugar. It is a gigantic myth that sugar is bad for you, because it does have beneficial properties. The bad stuff is highly refined white sugar. Natural sugar is a light to medium tan color and has a rich flavor. Low-Glycemic sugars raise your glucose levels slowly, so that your pancreas can process them without a blood sugar spike. This keeps you from feeling famished and exhausted after a meal.

Dark Raw Agave Syrup – This sugar is extracted from an agave plant, and is also used to make tequila. Agave is a rich sweet syrup but it doesn't harm your body the same way that refined sugar does. It is low glycemic, meaning it is high in fructose instead of glucose. Agave is great on pancakes, for baking and cooking, and added to teas. However, using agave daily isn't recommended. Your body can become dependent on the sweetness.

Raw Local Honey – Why raw and why local? Buying honey this way can help with allergies and provide an immune system boost. When it is raw and local the honey retains all of its nutrients and beneficial minerals. Honey is excellent on bread, in baked goods, added to tea and coffee, and so much more. Raw honey is delicious and nutritious, and doesn't spike blood sugar levels. This makes honey an excellent choice for those watching their sugar intake.

Coconut Sugar – This stuff may be hard to find for some, but it is sold at most health food and natural food stores. This sugar is produced with the sap from coconut flowers. Sweetness, flavor, and color will vary from package to package. However it resembles brown sugar and is perfect for baking or adding to foods you would fill with refined sugar. It is also considered a low-glycemic index food, high in iron, potassium, and other minerals.

Sucanat – This is pure evaporated cane juice. Nothing more than that, and nothing is taken away from it either. Sucanat is an excellent choice for baking delectable goods that are also diet friendly. While it isn't a "weight loss" tool, using sucanat in place of white refined sugar will keep blood sugar levels stable. Sucanat also contains all of the minerals and vitamins that sugar cane has. Sucanat is how sugar looks before it is refined into white sugar.

Artificial Sweeteners

If you are trying to lose weight there is a good chance that you have switched to artificial sweeteners. Diet soda, diet juices, sugar-free treats, even vitamin "water" contains artificial sweeteners. But what are they and why are they getting a bad reputation lately?

Artificial sweeteners are a sugar substitute that tastes sweet and acts like sugar where sugar would be used normally. Aspartame and Splenda are the most widely known artificial sugars that are added to just about every diet or sugar free food on the market. They add virtually 0 calories and taste very sweet once you get used to the flavor of them.

These artificial sugars are the most common:

Acesulfame Potassium – This artificial sweetener is said to be 180 to 200 times sweeter to the taste buds than regular refined white sugar. It is derived in part from potassium, as you could guess from the name. This sweetener is marketed as Sunett or Sweet One.

Aspartame – A chemical sweetener that is up for speculation on the safety of consumption. While it is generally seen as safe, there are some doubts about the true safety of consuming Aspartame. However, it is widely used in products like Diet Coke and Diet Pepsi, and other diet sodas. It is cheap and effective for making foods taste "sweet".

Saccharin – This sweetener is interesting because it is significantly sweeter than sugar but has an aftertaste that resembles something metallic and unpleasant. Most people do not enjoy saccharin but it is used to sweeten dozens of food products, especially toothpaste.

Sucralose – This sweetener is most commonly known as Splenda. While it is sold under different names, Splenda dominates the market. It is touted as the perfect sugar alternative for diabetics or those just trying to lose weight.

Splenda is relatively expensive for using as a regular replacement, but most people seem to like the flavor and ease of cooking with sucralose.

But are artificial sweeteners worth it? There are plenty of seemingly great benefits. Those trying to lose weight can replace refined white sugar with some artificially sweetened products and cut hundreds of calories. This is especially true for candy, ice cream, and sodas. Diabetics and those with insulin sensitivity have a lot to gain by making the switch to artificial sweeteners. However, many reports suggest that artificial sugars can lead to increased weight over the course of several years. Studies show those that regularly consume artificial sweeteners have bigger waist lines and are more likely to be overweight.

Another benefit of artificial sweeteners is that they do not cause tooth decay. However, the products that are often filled with artificial sugars do cause decay.

The dangers of artificial sweeteners apply to those that use them daily. Regular use of them causes dependence, irritable mood, a spiked craving for junk food, and yes, possible weight gain. Several studies have shown that individuals consuming aspartame or sucralose in higher doses, have an increased desire for sugary foods. This is because your brain realizes that the sweet flavor contains no actual sugar. You are not satisfying your bodies need to have a little sugar here and there, but instead you are silencing those cravings.

Dieters that are interested in using the artificial sweeteners mentioned above should do so in very limited quantities. Above all else, it is OK to have a little sugar here and there. In fact, any of the low glycemic sugars previously mentioned is safe, delicious, and actually healthy to consume in limited quantities. You can have your cake and eat it too!

Sugar Alcohols

Sugar alcohols are yet another choice in the world of sweetening food without all of the calories. Sugar alcohols occur naturally in foods such as fruits, vegetables, and grains. Corn is the most common grain used to extract sugar alcohols. These are used in sugar free chewing gum, candies, and sometimes beverages. They make a fantastic alternative to sugar and artificial sweeteners because they are natural and less caloric. Their taste is not as sweet as sugar.

- **Erythritol** – This is a food additive that has virtually 0 calories and is one of the lowest calorie sugar alcohols on the market. It is produced by fermentation process with yeast, and it occurs naturally in some fruits. It also does not cause tooth decay or weight problems. Best of all, it is the least likely to cause digestive disturbances after consuming food containing Erythritol.
- **Isomalt** – This tastes best when it is combined with another artificial sweetener. It is commonly used in many processed foods. It has some calories, but is still less than that of table sugar. Isomalt is not absorbed by the body so you may not digest or absorb all of the calories from it.
- **Lactitol** – One of the few sugar alcohols that is great for baking. It is very low in calories. Lactitol is used in medications and as a laxative, so use it with care.
- **Maltitol** – This is a very common sugar alcohol that is derived from corn. It is almost comparable to sugar, but is a tiny bit less sweet. It is found in

almost all chewing gum products and is seen as relatively safe to consume.

- **Mannitol** – An excellent choice for coating dried fruits and similar products, as it usually remains dry but sweet. It also does not increase blood glucose levels.
- **Sorbitol** – This sugar alcohol is found in apples, pears, and peaches. When consumed the body absorbs and digests it very slowly, making it ideal for those trying to lose weight or eat healthier.
- **Xylitol** – This is one of the best sugar alcohols on the market, as it works very well for baking and as a substitute all around. It is safe for the teeth and tastes great as well.
- **Stevia** – This relatively "new" sweetener is catching on around the country as the hottest new sweetener product to try. It is "natural" but also highly refined. It is considered very safe for use and one of the best choices for sweetening drinks and some foods. It is not recommended to bake with though, because it is still relatively pricey. Stevia has been approved for use in Diet Sodas like Coke and Pepsi for the end of 2011. It is widely available and adds a nice flavor to teas and coffee.

Sugar alcohols are a great choice if you can tolerate the minty cooling aftertaste. This is usually not noticeable, but some people notice the sensation and dislike the taste. Stevia also seems to cause allergic reactions for some people.

How to Use "Good" Sugar In Cooking

Before you get too excited and start cooking with all of these new-found sugar substitutes or healthier sugars, do your research. An entire book could be filled describing the many ways to use these sugars for cooking baked goods, meals, and making drinks. However they are not as common as regular sugar so variances will happen. When you are preparing meals with substitutes it is important to know how each sugar works.

Agave nectar for example, should be used in a smaller amount than regular table sugar. You would not use 1 cup of agave instead of 1 cup of sugar. Instead you would go for a half cup to 3/4ths cup. This will provide adequate sweetness.

Honey works the same way, and using too much can lead to a very sticky and gooey product at the end of cooking.

Sucanat is a 1 to 1 ratio for cooking. If the recipe calls for 1 cup of sugar, use 1 cup of sucanat. This applies for all sugars like coconut sugar too.

Sugar alcohols usually require more to make it the desired sweetness, and some do not cook very well at all. For each individual alcohol you should go on a case by case basis. Even better would be to find recipes that specifically use these sugar alcohols, so that no mistakes can be made.

Once you learn to cook with alternatives to refined sugar, you will be healthier and realize that living a healthy lifestyle free from refined sugars is easy and tastes just as good.

Adding Whole Grains to Your Diet
Whole grains cannot be stressed enough, as they are so immensely important to overall health and vitality. Adding grains is easy, cheap, and delicious.

For breakfast you can try whole grain cereals. Look for sugar free types or those with less than 8 grams of sugar per serving. These cereals are usually packed with at least 20 grams of whole grains, tons of fiber, and even some protein to keep you full for long periods of time.

Toast and whole grain bread is also a great option. Look for brands that do not use enriched flours. If the bread has wheat, spelt, barley, and oats, it is probably a healthy choice. Many whole wheat products contain refined white flour as well, so always check your label.

Whole grain pasta can be difficult to work with, especially since they cook slightly different from white pasta. However, whole grain pasta is just as affordable and delicious as the normal kind. They come with more nutrients, fiber, and protein. You may also find yourself eating less whole wheat pasta than refined, because it makes you full faster.

Corn tortillas are a surprisingly excellent way to add a nutritious whole grain to your diet. Not only are corn tortillas smaller, but they have more flavor than white flour tortillas.

When baking, opt for oatmeal and whole wheat flour. Cakes and muffins taste just as good with healthier ingredients as their sugary refined carbohydrate counterparts. Your kids and family members won't know the difference.

Air popped pop corn makes an excellent snack. Lightly coat with coconut oil and you have a sweet and salty snack that has fiber and is low in calories!

Dealing with Food Allergies

Food allergies are annoying and make eating anything difficult, especially with multiple sensitivities and problems. When it comes to losing weight while eating a diet void of your allergens, you may feel angry and frustrated at the limited options available. The food industry is becoming more aware of the problems facing those with allergies, and is accommodating the needs of many with creative food products that aid in weight loss and keep you feeling healthy.

Peanut Allergies

Most foods are processed with peanut allergies in mind. It is fairly simple and straightforward, just avoid peanuts. Most nut butters are processed in factories where peanuts are also processed. If this is a problem for you, read every label and send in emails when necessary.

Lactose Sensitivity and Milk Allergies

Milk is in everything it seems, and once you think you found a product without milk – you realize it has it. Look for certified vegan products and avoid the following ingredients:

- Artificial butter flavor
- Artificial coffee creamers
- Casein (or any ingredient that includes this word or "caseinate")
- Caseinates
- Custard
- Ghee
- Hydrolysates
- Kefir

- Koumiss
- Lactalbumin
- Lactalbumin phosphate
- Lactoglobulin
- Lactose
- Lactulose
- Nougat
- Paneer
- Potasium Caseinate
- Pudding
- Rennet casein
- Whey

These are just a few examples, but once you familiarize yourself with these terms and foods that contain dairy, you can easily avoid upsetting your body by consuming those products.

There are plenty of replacements that are excellent for cooking and baking too, so you won't have to miss out totally. You can find soy milk, almond milk, oat milk, hemp, and other replacements with minimal difficulty. Ice creams and cheeses are usually made with alternative ingredients too, making substitutions in your meals fast, easy, and healthier than their "real" counterparts in many cases.

Gluten Allergies

A number of people are developing Celiac disease and have other problems when it comes to consuming gluten. Gluten is found in any wheat or grain product, including oats, wheat bread, flours, and even candies. Gluten ends up in skincare and hair care products too. With gluten free awareness on the rise, there are dozens of pastas and breads made with gluten free ingredients. There are even cookies and muffins designed for the person with a gluten allergy. You can find these online and at health food stores. Even big box grocery stores are starting to stock gluten free products, so that you can enjoy a small bowl of fettuccine with tomato sauce too.

Soy Allergies

This is an allergen that encompasses more foods than any other on the market. Soy is used in literally every food product you can imagine, in some way. Avoiding soy in your diet can help you lose weight if you have an allergy. There are no guidelines to what specific products to avoid, but you must be diligent about reading labels. Eating soy-free will require preparing almost all of your meals at home and from scratch. While this seems complicated to do, you will likely end up dropping weight as a result of this dramatic change.

Removing soy from your diet is a lot easier when you make food from scratch. Many cookbooks will offer soy free meal ideas. A soy free diet is possible, even as a vegetarian. You just need more grains, nuts, fruits, and vegetables.

2.3 - Foods That Have a Negative Impact On Your Health

Before you get into this section, please remember that these are only guidelines. The goal is not to become obsessed with perfection, but rather, improve everything you possibly can. Not everyone can make immediate changes in one day and switch their entire way of life. It is not financially feasible to do so, and your taste buds may not be happy if you do. Of course, if you are able to drop everything and overhaul your lifestyle, by all means do that. You will be happier once you try.

Frozen Meals

When you are trying to lose weight, frozen meals can seem like the easiest route to take. They are moderately cheap, they taste OK, and they seem to provide the right amount of nutrition. The fact of the matter is that, frozen meals are your worst enemy. Avoid them. If you really like certain ones, make it from scratch! Many frozen meals are pasta based or pizza based. These two things are easy to make on your own for less money and better overall nutrition. Plus you control the amount of salt that goes in and stays out of your body.

Also consider that frozen foods can contain toxic chemicals leeched into the product when microwaving. Many ready to heat and eat packages use BPA and other chemicals to produce the plastic and cardboard. When in doubt, opt for organic and natural frozen foods. There are plenty that use high quality simple ingredients, without all of the junk your body doesn't need.

A much nicer option to try out is creating your own frozen meals. By simply cooking some of your favorite healthy meals in advance, you can create quick to prepare frozen meals by sorting out some portions onto a microwave safe dish which you can cover with cellophane wrap, let cool then eventually freeze. This is best accomplished using a freezer with a deep freeze option to allow for longer storage. To reheat your homemade frozen meals all you have to do is take them out and thaw them using a microwave.

Note: Certain starchy foods will generally not reheat as well from a frozen state. Take for instance, pastas or potatoes which have been frozen may reconstitute as a mushy byproduct rather than their original forms. It is a great idea to experiment with different dishes to ensure that they can reheat well once frozen to make note of for future freezing options. This can even be tested on leftovers of particularly favorite meal options that you have created recently.

This method of preparing your own frozen meals not only helps to save you money on the materials to create the meals, but you also reduce the number of toxic chemicals that are put into your food once they are prepared. Since you will not be using preservatives or other harmful additives in your foods, you will also reduce the work load of your vital organs such as your liver, kidneys and gallbladder.

Candy
For the most part, candies are a waste of calories and money. They provide absolutely nothing beneficial for the body. Laying off the candy alone will likely help you drop a few pounds right away. There are some instances where candy is all right, such as eating dark chocolate. A small piece of dark chocolate, usually less than 1 ounce, contains iron and antioxidants.

Candy alternatives are always the way to go when you are trying to change to a healthier lifestyle which incorporates weight loss. A great alternative to candy is having naturally sweetened foods such as organic raisins which have been sun-ripened and dried. You can find a wide variety of fruits and even vegetables which become sweeter once they have been dehydrated which will leave behind naturally occurring, low glycemic fructose sugars while creating a chewy and interactive piece of food which is also delicious.

Canned Foods

These seem like a good choice because they are shelf stable and cheap. But buying all of your beans, vegetables, fruits, and meals from the canned isle is a bad idea. Even so-called light vegetable soups offer you almost nothing in terms of nutrition. In fact, many light soups targeted to dieters contain less than fresh quality vegetables, chicken stock, and about 120 calories per can. These soups usually sell for $2 per can, while non-diet targeted soups are $1 per can and have double the calories. Essentially you are paying a premium price for less food and thus, less nutrition.

How do you fix this problem? Purchase frozen fruits and vegetables instead. They are frozen during their peak and taste great when steamed or blended into smoothies. Make soup from scratch and leave it in a crock pot to cook for the entire day which blends the flavors to create a simple yet delicious meal which can also be portioned out and stored for later via freezing.

Energy Drinks and Sports Drinks

When someone starts an exercise program it is natural to think that you need energy drinks and sports drinks. The facts are, if you are exercising less than 1 hour per day at a low to moderate intensity, then no additional drinks are needed. If you drink sports drinks while doing this, you will likely just set yourself back and end up gaining weight or stalling at the same weight for a long period of time.

If you are exercising at a moderate to high intensity for over 1 hour, then it is all right to choose a sugar free and low calorie sports drink. Leave caffeine out of the mix, as it will fatigue your muscles more than it will help.

Energy drinks are not necessarily bad when they are natural, sugar free, and low in caffeine. But many commercial drinks on the market contain too much caffeine and sugars to make them worth using for weight loss or energy during your workouts. Try finding organic and non-sweetened energy drinks which use alternatives to sugars and caffeine to keep you going.

"Healthy" Fast Food Meals
It's true that you can eat decently on the go without ruining your entire daily fast food budget. But most fast food meals, even when marketed as healthy, contain too many calories. You will likely want fries with that too, which are an empty calorie bomb to your day.

For smart ordering on the go, aim for the freshest foods on the menu. McDonald's has great premium salads with grilled chicken, and you can order without the chicken as well. Fast food restaurants have a habit of giving you the dressing that "goes with" the salad choice, but if it is a high calorie or unhealthy option, simply ask for a different one to suit your needs.

Grilled chicken sandwiches are a safe bet, but only if you skip the mayo and cheese. Use half a bun, since fast food buns are usually dense and contain a lot of calories and minimal fiber. If you must order fries, share with someone or get a small order instead.

Unsweetened teas are the perfect drink for a meal on the go, but if that isn't available, always opt for water instead. Most places offer water for free, so you save a few dollars too.

2.4 - Supplementing Your Diet

Diet supplementation is a popular trend that is taking over the health food industry. Every corner you look there is a company pleading with consumers to purchase their products that are a "miracle" cure for weight loss or health. Supplements can be great for you but it is important to know which ones are necessary, and which ones probably won't help at all.

Let's take Acai berry pills for example. These pills promise to make you shed weight and build strong muscles in no time at all. Juices and powders fill shelves of grocery stores, all with the promise of making you a healthier person. The Acai berry is delicious and packed with antioxidants, but it isn't any more special than blueberries. Acai is just another exotic berry that cannot be shipped to the United States. Acai supplements are a scam, and you shouldn't take them for weight loss.

Multi-vitamins are a good choice though, especially if you are on a restricted calorie diet. It may be difficult to get all of the vitamins and minerals you need. A multi-vitamin will give you that extra boost to keep your vitamin levels steady. If you happen to take in more vitamins than needed, that's fine too.

If you are feeling lethargic or tired, a multi-vitamin may be the answer.

Omega-3 supplements are also 100% necessary. Most people do not get enough omega-3 in their diet. The American diet is full of omega-6 fats, which are also known as polyunsaturated fats. If you have an improper balance of omega-3 to omega-6, it could result in a number of health problems. However, 1 daily pill of 1,000 mg of omega-3 is enough to balance your body. After 6 weeks of consistent use, you will feel stronger, healthier, and more alert. It preserves the brain, lowers cholesterol and increases good cholesterol, and makes the skin radiant. An important note to add is that omega-3 fish oil can be risky. Be sure your fish oil is from toxin free fish and does not contain shark. Pure salmon from the Northwest Pacific is your best choice. If this isn't a possibility, go for flaxseed oil pills. There is less risk for toxicity and your body converts it to DHA.

Diet pills are generally not recommended. However, in some instances they can be acceptable. Alli for example, is approved by the FDA and numerous people have had success using this as part of a weight loss plan. Many diet pills are really just vitamins and energizers in high doses. For example, B-vitamins provide a lot of energy to the body and if you take over 1,000% of your Daily Value, you will feel very energetic. This is safer than high caffeine pills or drinks. Read labels and know what you are considering taking before you do so.

HCG is a new trend, involving pregnancy hormones and weight loss. It requires that you eat only 500 calories per day and take shots or drinks with HCG. This diet fad is a huge scam and will not help you lose weight in a healthy manner.

Anything that involves "hormones" is probably dangerous and not worth the extremely high cost.

Muscle supplement powders are also a hot trend for men. Unless you intend to body build for competition and profession, step away from the muscle supplements. They are unnecessary and expensive for the average person trying to simply lose weight and gain muscle.

Protein supplements on the other hand, can be beneficial when used sparingly. Most powders, such as whey, contain a whopping 40 grams of protein per serving. This is almost your entire daily need for protein. Go with one-fourth or half of that to get a healthy amount of protein added in. You can mix protein supplement with fruit or vegetable smoothies, or even mix it in oatmeal for a little extra boost.

Other health pills can also be taken to boost your body in areas where you may be lacking. For example, Gingko Balboa is shown to improve cognitive function and memory. Taking supplements of herbs and plants can be beneficial, but be sure to educate yourself on each individual one beforehand. Some may cause allergic reactions.

2.5 - Juicing and Green Smoothies
Part of a healthy diet is eating plenty of green vegetables and fruits, which was thoroughly covered earlier. Juicing and green smoothies are a tasty way to chug your recommended three cups of green vegetables per week, and possibly get many more than that in your diet.

Juicing has proven benefits, such as raw consumption of pure vegetables. You get the vitamins and minerals in a few swigs, instead of chopping your way through a plate full of greens. You can sweeten juices with fruit to make them more palatable too.

Juicing will help with weight loss by boosting vitamin levels and providing energy to the body to burn fat. Fruits and veggies, particularly leafy greens, are substantial when it comes to getting your body all the nutrients that it needs.

Smoothies are a little creamier and usually contain more fruit. If you are new to juicing and green smoothies, use 1/4 cup of greens to start, and 3/4 cup of fruit. You may also add in low fat yogurt and skim milk or a milk alternative.

As you get used to drinking so much nutrition in one cup, you can increase the amount of veggies you use. Your body may not tolerate so much at once, resulting in vomiting or other discomfort. Working up to including more veggies is the best way for your body to tolerate it.

Why does juicing and green smoothies promote weight loss? The best guess that dieticians offer is that they are packed with so many nutrients and fiber in one meal, that your metabolism is revved. If you drink a green concoction you will notice increased energy and fullness and a healthier overall outlook for the day.

2.6 - Food Measurements – What Is An Appropriate Portion Size?

Now that you have learned new information about food and what kind of foods to eat, you need to learn more about portion sizes. The world of serving sizes is complicated and at some points, very frustrating. In many cases you run into situations where the exact amount is undefined and hard to imagine or use. Aside from tablespoons versus teaspoons, cup, and half cup, what about all of the other stuff like gram weights?

When you make this lifestyle change you are going to want to learn grams. Beside every package of food the nutrition label will say something like:

"1 Serving (140 grams)"

That's all they tell you! Well, is that one piece or two? A half cup or one fourth? See how complicated things can get? This is where a food scale becomes of big importance, especially when weighing natural whole foods. It's difficult to count calories and record your food if you do not know how much you are eating.

Instead of guessing, buy a set of measurement cups. They are cheap and a great weight loss tool. You should also purchase dipped tablespoon and teaspoon measuring spoons. These will give you a more accurate measurement than if you were to use a regular tablespoon made for eating.

A food scale can measure in ounces and grams and is very sensitive for food products. To measure your food, place your plate on the scale, then tare. You can then pile on each individual food you are going to consume, and tare after each placement.

If you are weighing a homemade taco for instance, you would place the tortilla, tare, then place the filling, tare, veggies, tare, and then cheese or sour cream toppings. Write down each measurement in grams and calculate the total calories online. This method is fast and effective, because you get the exact amount of food you need, without overindulging by accident.

If you weigh your food but have no idea how many calories it contains, an online calorie tracker is usually able to help you. If you don't know the nutrition of dried mango, you can find a generic listing, input the gram weight, and get all the information you need. Natural foods are usually the same in nutrition so weighing is the best way to determine what is in your food nutrition-wise.

When you don't have a scale or other measuring tools to go by, you must judge based on eyeballing your food measurements. Most of these eyeball measurements are compared to a physical object that most people will recognize in their head to get an idea of a product weight.

One ounce of a grain is about the size of a plastic CD case. This includes cereal, rice, pasta, and breads. 2 servings would be about the size of a tennis ball. The tennis ball measurement is more accurate for rice and other loose grain food measurements.

Vegetables will vary since they are all different shapes and sizes. In general 1 serving of vegetables is a half cup cooked. One half cup of potato is the size of a standard computer mouse.

Fruit servings are usually one full fruit as long as it is a medium size. Giant fruits are going to be multiple servings. One fruit serving would be the size of a standard tennis ball, while cut fruit would equal the amount of 7 cotton ball sizes. So that means 7 large grapes or 7 cubes of melon.

Dairy is varied. One serving is 1 cup of milk, up to 2 ounces of cheese, or 1.5 cups of ice cream. If low fat options are not available where you are eating, choose smaller portion sizes. One serving of cheese is the size of two die in cubes or two 9-volt batteries.

The protein group is also complicated. One ounce is one protein serving of lean meat, poultry, fish, or tofu. You can have up to 4 ounces of these per day so choose wisely. A serving of fish is about 1 checkbook size. A serving of meat or poultry is 1 deck of cards sized, or palm sized. Everyone's palm is a different size but go by your own. Two servings of peanut butter will be about a ping pong ball size for two tablespoons. Nuts and seeds are a half ounce per serving so it will usually be a small handful size.

When choosing dressing from salad bars you should be careful with portion sizes. Most dressing ladles are 1/4 cup to 1/2 cup in size! This can add hundreds of calories depending on the dressing you choose. To be safe go for Italian, light ranch, and vinaigrette dressing. Put your dressing in a separate dish. When you eat your salad, don't pour your dressing on top. Instead, dip your fork lightly in your dish of dressing. This provides a perfect measurement for what you need.

2.7 - Meal Planning
If you subscribe to any health magazines or have read a diet book at least once in your life, you would know that meal planning is a vital part of "dieting." Planning your meals to reflect your health needs each day is an excellent way to stay on track and incorporate variety and interesting food into your life. Meal planning can take some time but once you are

used to the idea you will find that it comes fast and is almost like second nature.

Effective meal planning begins with having an idea. What kind of foods do you enjoy? Do you like ethnic food like Mexican and Chinese? Search for recipes in your favorite cookbooks or online, and decide what meal you want to cook those recipes for. Organizing 7 dinners, 7 lunches, and 7 breakfasts per week is easy and fun. If you like consistency you can even eat the same thing each day, but that isn't recommended.

Try to choose a high fiber and high protein breakfast with fruit, a lunch with ample veggies and light lean protein, and a dinner that is small but satisfying. Desserts and snacks can be included too, as long as your calorie budget allows for it!

Write down what foods you want to cook for each day of the week, using recipes or just basic meal ideas. Figure out how much of certain foods you will need that week, and write them down for your grocery list. A good grocery list should have plenty of fruits and vegetables and grains, a small amount of lean meat, and a very small amount of processed foods.

If you need help with meal planning, thumb through magazines to see how they arrange their diet plans. Take ideas that you think would taste good, and put those for your own. You don't need to follow those plans exactly, because they rarely suit everyone's budget or tastes. The plan is to be inspired by other meal plan sources.

Meal planning can become tiresome. So save all of your plans for each week and repeat them each month. This works great because you won't have the same thing until the next month, but you get plenty of diversity and healthy foods in your diet. This keeps your body satisfied with what you are feeding it, and energized to help you shed pounds.

2.8 - Food Preparation/Storage

One thing that dieters often complain about when it comes to food preparation is time and storage. Most people do not know how to prepare healthy meals and then save it for later. Busy adults that work may find that it is easier to do a drive through run instead of taking 30 minutes to make a healthy meal for themselves and or their family.

A good trick is to prepare a few meals on a free day, such as Sunday. Make soups, stews, even healthy burgers. After preparing your lunches or dinners for the week, you can weigh them and portion them out into individual storage containers. Most foods can be refrigerated for 3 days but you should freeze food for later in the week. Take out your prepared food when you want to have it for a meal and eat. You save a lot of time preparing food in bulk, especially when the work week gets hectic with schedules and deadlines.

You can usually purchase storage containers that are BPA free and freezer safe for less than $30 for a large set. They come in portion controlled sizes from a half cup to several cups.

Deep Freezing and Dehydrating Fresh Food

Another trick that experts use is to deep freeze or dehydrate fresh foods. Fruits and vegetables, as well as some fresh grains, often go bad at a very rapid pace. In the winter there isn't a wide variety of fruit available, as most fruits are spring and summer. When fruit is in season, buy as much of it as possible. You can usually chop it and deep freeze to use when the fruit season is over, and you save tons of money by not purchasing something like blueberries for $5 a per small pint or half pint!

There are tips and tricks for deep freezing, but a good rule of thumb is to always wash your produce thoroughly before freezing. You may also want to cut off stems, remove seeds or pits, and toss out any blemished fruits. One fruit you should avoid freezing is pineapple. The reason behind this is that pineapple tends to taste bitter and less sweet after freezing. Grapes, strawberries, raspberries, blueberries, and diced mango are great options for deep freezing. For vegetables, you can freeze spinach at the peak of harvest, as it gets more expensive during off seasons. Use frozen spinach in pasta and baked dishes when it gets chilly outside.

Dehydrating fresh food is a little different. These will be more for snacking and not cooking. You can make raisins and cranberries as well as dried blueberries for oatmeal. A quality dehydrator is a great investment.

After you have dried and dehydrated your food you should use them within 6 months. While dehydrating does stop them from rotting, without the sophisticated technology that food processing plants use, you cannot ensure that they will last longer than 6 months.

Using this method you can have fresh food even during the long cold months where quality produce is hard to come by. The benefits include more variety in your diet, delicious fruits you crave out of season, and plenty of vitamins too.

2.9 - Food Logs

Now that you have read this comprehensive section on healthy eating, how to plan and prepare food, and suggestions for healthy serving sizes, how do you put it all together? Food logs are consistently proven to be the #1 weight loss tool. Food diaries keep you in check by recording your entire intake and showing the potential flaws in your dieting for the day. Food diaries hold you accountable for what you eat, and make it easy to track exactly what went into your mouth.

Better yet, food logs are great to print off and show to your doctor during checkups. That way you can show how you have been eating the last few weeks or months, and the doctor can determine what your next step should be for good health and weight loss.

If you prefer to write on paper, a good journal is a great resource for keeping track of food. You can transport it anywhere and write down what you eat and revisit the journal later. Or you can sign up for one of the many free online services such as www.sparkpeople.com, where you can get very detailed daily reports and keep track of every last gram of food.

Online databases are sometimes incorrect when you choose a food. Some may say that a small order of McDonald's fries has 400 calories, when it really has about 280 calories. For this reason you should cross check every food you input to be sure it is accurate. Using a site like Spark People, you can input your own recipes, foods, favorites, and more. They are saved to your account so you can just click and input for your meals that day. It makes logging your food fast, easy, and efficient.

Even better, you can access Spark People from any device with an internet connection. There are even Smartphone apps that you can use to input your food intake while traveling or on the go. There are no excuses for not logging your food with the technology available today. The countless applications for food diaries are great if you eat out a lot or dine at a friend's house.

Food tracking is an excellent tool, and if you follow it daily you will find that it is easy to do naturally. It may be time consuming when you first start, but after a few weeks of doing it each day you will become an expert at inputting your food for the day. You may even find it enjoyable and a nice way to wind down at the end of a stressful day. Comprehensive reports can show if you ate too much sodium or lacked in protein, so that you can fix it the next day. With food logging there is no room for failure, as you are always being aware of what goes in your mouth.

3 - Exercise

Exercise is a necessary evil in weight loss that most people will protest to at least once on their journey. Not everyone has a problem with exercise which makes it much easier to accomplish once the process has started. Consulting your doctor before starting an exercise regimen is also necessary to help you understand what types of exercises should be avoided, especially if you have any extraneous conditions which may make certain exercises dangerous for you. This precaution is well recommended at least until you are able to safely do them once you have progressed.

How to Start an Exercise Program

Let's pretend that you have never exercised a day in your life. Pretend that you are starting from scratch completely. Forget all that you know and all that you have done in the past. Think of a goal that you want to achieve, and plot what exercises you enjoy doing the most. Do you prefer fast walking? Are you a runner or a cyclist? Do you prefer gym classes led by an instructor? Do you like to take it to the hills and hike? Or would you feel more in your element by swimming in a pool for your workouts? Whatever you enjoy doing, do more of it. This section will elaborate on ideas to get you into the mood for exercising by starting slow and then going big. After all, Rome wasn't built in a day.

Building a Walking Regimen

They say that walking 6 miles per week at a minimum will strengthen brain tissue and help you retain memory over the course of your life. Walking boosts gray matter while providing a low-impact fun exercise. To start a walking program be sure that you have cushioned shoes and comfortable clothes. There are several sources online that allow you to plan your routes precisely so that you know how much mileage you are doing.

After you plan your route, start by walking it once per day, seven days per week. It is best to start with just one mile so that you can work up to doing it more frequently. One mile per day is sufficient enough for a beginner. You may also want to purchase walking sticks. They lower the impact on your joints as you walk, while increasing your calorie burn rate by about 40%.

Walking is the easiest exercise for beginners. Before each walk warm up by stretching your knees and ankles. Bend side to side to loosen up the body. This will help your muscles adapt to walking.

After you are no longer a beginner walker, you can increase the intensity of your exercise. At this point it might be a good idea to add in wrist or ankle weights. You will create more resistance to fuel the burn. Carrying a backpack with weights inside is also an excellent way to make walking more of a challenge.

When one mile becomes too easy, increase it to 1.5 miles per day. Every two weeks after the first month you can increase your mileage by a half mile. Your workout should look like this:

First Month: 1 mile per day

Week 5: 1.5 miles per day

Week 6: 1.5 miles per day

Week 7: 2 miles per day

Week 8: 2 miles per day

Continue this pattern until you reach a specific mileage goal for your walking routine.

Building a Running Routine

Novice runners should start with the beginner walking program first. While it may begin to seem slow near the end, stick with walking before you run. Running can be exhilarating and freeing but if you go too fast too soon you will likely injure your knees or ankles.

A running routine requires dedication and diligence. This is a sample plan you can follow that you will help you become a steady strong runner within two months time, as well as burn off extra fat. Keep in mind that your weight and size are not as important when it comes to running. The important thing is that you have proper form and skill for the task you are about to take on.

To prepare your body for a running routine, you must start by running twice per week for 4 weeks. Use the trail you follow for walking and instead of walking two days, run the route at a comfortable pace. After 1 month of running twice per week, it is safe to increase that number to 3 days per week.

It is important to do interval training as well. Not only will it torch calories as you train, but you will gain speed and get faster as you go. Interval training can be done like this:

Run for 3 minutes at medium pace.

Slow to a comfortable pace for 1 minute.

Increase to a faster running pace for 2 minutes.

Repeat as often as you would like. Interval training is unique because there is something for anyone. There are no specific speeds to follow. The goal is to challenge your body to the limit then rest and bring yourself back up. When you keep your body guessing you burn more calories.

Other Workout Methods for Starting Slow and Building Strong
Running and walking are the two core workouts that people aim for when it comes down to losing weight, but there are a number of other workouts you can do to keep your body

going strong by the day. Weight training is a crucial way to build bone density and lean muscle mass. Cross training is important as well, so that your body doesn't burn out and stop responding to your exercise routines.

Tips to Gain Strength:

- Exercise consistently. Taking frequent breaks will not help you get stronger in the long run.

- Be sure to hydrate and consume enough balanced meals to fuel your muscles.

- If you feel exhausted, listen to your body and take a rest day or do light exercise on a resting day.

- Cross train. This means instead of walking every single day, and doing nothing else, incorporate a different exercise or piece of equipment on top of your routine. Your muscles will have to keep guessing.

- Use interval training. Find a method for intervals that works for your goals and stick with it for two weeks, then change to a new interval routine.

Calculating Calories Burned For Optimum Weight Loss
So you are working out on a regular basis, and you think you are at the right intensity. But how can you be sure you are working hard enough to burn the right amount of calories? Gym machines are accurate to a certain degree, but most require that you keep your hands on the sensors at all times. This can be a hassle. Some machines do not account for your

age, gender, weight, and height. This also skews the accuracy of the amount of calories burned.

The best method for determining how much you are burning is by using a heart rate monitor. An HRM uses a strap that goes around your chest and uses sensors to monitor your heart rate. This is consistent because it is always in contact with your skin. This device relays information to a watch that you wear, and keeps you updated on your current heart rate. The HRM does the calculations that include your height, weight, age, and gender, to determine an approximate amount of calories burned.

When you have a more accurate number you can better gauge what your intake should be. Most people grossly overestimate the amount of calories they burn during their exercise routines.

Exercising Safely

When you start an exercise program you should always ask your doctor for advice on what is safe for your body. If you have health restrictions get more information on what will benefit you most. Walking is usually the safest bet for any beginner, but if you want diversity you will need to take extra precautions to prevent injury.

Stretching before your workouts will be beneficial. Limber up and do what feels natural to your body. Stretch sideways, stretch your hamstrings, and do a few jumping jacks. This will prepare your body for the task at hand.

After exercising you should stretch as well. Frequent stretching will help prevent injury by reducing the amount of strain your muscles and tendons go through.

Never push yourself too hard. Over exertion can cause injury and pain. You can increase the intensity but if you feel a sharp pang anywhere in your body, it is time to slow down and finish up. Going for something you know your body cannot accomplish is setting yourself up for potential injury risk.

If you do happen to injure yourself, ice it with a compress and elevate it for as long as possible. Avoid intense exercise for a few days after an injury. If the problems last for more than a week or two, then see a doctor to evaluate what the problem is.

3.1 - The Importance of Exercise
Exercise is an absolute necessity to maintain good health and a strong body. Without physical activity your muscles almost disappear, your bones weaken, and you are susceptible to diseases and illness. Exercise regularly, even if it is just something small, because your body will thank you in the long run.

This may seem a bit obvious, but exercise controls your weight. When you exercise daily for 30 minutes or more, at a moderate intensity, you are helping your body fight off extra fat. The more you do the more you burn. To calculate your calorie burn accurately, it is recommended that you purchase a heart rate monitor. When you input your age, gender, weight, and height, it can give you an approximate amount of calories burned during your exercise. More so, it will let you know if you are working hard enough to shed the extra pounds. A good heart rate range to aim for is 130 beats per minute to 170 beats per minute. These numbers are averages and can vary depending on your age, experience with exercise, and ability to raise your heart rate.

Exercise also combats diabetes. When blood sugar levels are elevated, a burst of moderate activity will help return blood sugar levels to normal. Regular exercise for 20 minutes or more per day is shown to help blood sugar levels stay stabilized, even if you happen to enjoy a small treat. Instead of chaotic glucose levels, you will remain in the normal range.

Regular exercise also combats high blood pressure. It prevents and reduces the strain because your heart becomes efficient at controlling blood pressure levels. Plus you sweat out excess salts that encourage hypertension. Exercise works as both a prevention tool and a cure.

Activities at a low-impact state will increase good cholesterol while lowering bad cholesterol. The more you move the better it gets. Duration for this matters more than the intensity, so if you walk for 2 hours a day you will notice a big difference in your blood tests the next time you visit your doctor.

Additional health benefits include decreased depression, arthritis prevention, boosted moods, stronger bones, metabolic balance, and healthier skin. Just be sure to wear sun block if you exercise outdoors.

If you constantly feel tired and lethargic, exercise is the answer. A simple walk or jog will boost energy levels and productivity. Instead of drinking coffee in the morning, try a brisk walk. You will notice a better mood the entire day.

Sleep problems are often cured by proper exercise as well. If you work out hard in the morning, you will likely sleep like a baby that night. Exercise relaxes that body and puts it in a normal cycle of sleep. Poor diet and lack of exercise contribute to lethargy. Of course, exercising late at night is likely to cause insomnia. So exercise mid-day or early morning if possible.

If you are never "in the mood" then start exercising. Things like yoga and Pilates boost your sensitivity and make intimate encounters feel better. It boosts desire and happiness, which all lead to a better sex life. Better sex means a better relationship with your partner. This is healthy in a number of ways, so exercise and then reap the benefits.

There is a lot of fun to be had once you get in the habit of regular exercise. You can bond with your family or a close buddy, enjoy nature, and appreciate the things you couldn't before. There are few things more powerful-feeling than hiking a challenging trail at a state park or trekking to see a beautiful waterfall. The world opens up to you once you start exercising and gaining the strength to carry your body to new heights.

3.2 - Effective Exercise
If you want to lose weight you need to participate in activities that are effective for weight loss. One would assume that all exercise is effective, but this simply isn't true for the majority of people trying to shed stubborn fat and develop a lean body. The right amount of intensity matters as well as frequency and how your technique is.

Body Toning and Strengthening Exercises
Cardiovascular activity is only one small part of losing weight. While cardiovascular activities are necessary to burn fat and raise your metabolism, it is only one small piece of the equation. To effectively lose weight you must incorporate body toning exercises. This means incorporating resistance training, weight lifting, and plyometric exercises.

Why body tone? First of all, if you are overweight chances are you have a high body fat percentage as well. This isn't true for all overweight individuals, but for most it will be the case. Body fat is significantly more important than your BMI number. This is because fat can squeeze your organs, which is also known as visceral fat. This type of fat harms the organs in your abdominal region. It is the most dangerous type of fat to have, and is what usually causes heart attacks and other health related problems. This is why you want to do body toning exercises. When you build muscle your body burns off that excess fat trapped in and around your abdominal region.

Strength Training For Beginners
It's always an appropriate time to start strength training. You do not need to wait until your body is accustomed to cardio activity. However, it is very important that you start off slow, especially if you have never picked up a weight a day in your life. Strength training builds bone strength, muscle and tendon strength, increases your metabolism, and gives you a lean streamlined appearance.

The first 6 to 8 weeks of strength training you will really want to focus on your form and what works for you. Form is the #1 thing to pay attention to when you are getting into a strength-training routine. Slouching, bending the wrong way, or over-extending can lead to injury.

Start off by choosing a move to do for each area of your body. Arms, legs, buttocks, abdominal, and shoulder muscles are the ones you want to work. Most routines involve your entire body, so you don't have to worry too much about it. Choosing a video for beginners may also help you develop a program that you can use to strength train.

It is ideal to do this three times per week. You may strength train more frequently if you desire but over working your muscles will result in fatigue and a slow-down of muscle progress. To perform this routine you will need a set of light dumbbells ranging from 5 to 10 pounds, a stable seating surface or body ball, and a cushioned mat if you do not have a cushioned floor.

Floor Squats – Do one set of 12 reps. Be sure to keep your back very straight and do not bend your knees past your ankles. Over bending your knees will result in injuries to both the knee tendons as well as your ankles. Focus on slow precise movements.

Assisted Lunges – Do one set of 12 reps per leg. Holding a wall or stable surface, bend your right knee into a 90 degree position while bringing your left knee to the ground. Do not let your knee extend past your toe. Push your body back to a standing position, and repeat with the opposite leg. Lunges are difficult for beginners, so using a stable strong surface will help you complete assisted lunges safely and while strengthening your muscles.

Wall Pushups – Do one set of 12. If you are unable to perform a regular pushup or modified pushup, wall pushups are an excellent version that will give you upper body strength. Place your hands on a wall or strong surface. Straighten your back with legs together in a semi-relaxed position. Bend elbows as if you were doing a pushup on the floor, and then push back up. It is the same as a floor pushup, but since you are using a wall or strong surface, you can balance your body and use proper form. This exercise has all of the benefits of a push up, without the risk of injury to your shoulders, back, or wrists.

One-Armed Row – Do one set of 12 per arm. To do a one-armed row you hold your weight of choice in your left hand and place your right hand on the right thigh. Bend as straight as possible so that it looks as if you are bending over to pick something off the floor. Lift the weight in your left hand up, bending your elbow toward you. Lower slowly and repeat. This move works your lateral muscles and biceps.

Lateral Raises – Do one set of 12. Get into a rigid standing position. Shoulders back, spine aligned, and legs hip-width apart. Use two dumbbells of your weight choice, one in each hand – 5 pounds each or 2.5 pounds each is recommended. Do not lock your elbows, but leave them slightly bent. Lift arms to your sides, straight out, and hold for 2 seconds. Lower your arms slowly, then repeat. This move works your shoulders and arms.

Hammer Curls – Do one set of 12. Stand with your feet the traditional hip-width apart. Keep your posture straight. If you have difficulty keeping a straight posture, sitting in a rigid chair may be beneficial. Hold your dumbbells with your hands facing each other at your hips. Then bend your arms up at a loose 90 degree angle so that your dumbbells are facing each other at chest level. Lower slowly, then repeat.

Tricep Extensions – Do one set of 12 reps per arm. This is a very easy move that is great for sitting exercises. Hold a light weight in one arm. Lift your arm so that your elbow is bent and positioned at the side of your head. Take your opposite free hand and hold your elbow steady. Lower the weight behind your head, and then lift as if you were stretching to the ceiling. This move is extremely easy but you will feel the burn after 12 reps. Repeat with opposite arm.

Seated Rotations – Do one set of 12 complete rotations. Instead of traditional crunches, seated rotations offer a comfortable position that is still effective for abdominal exercises. To do this move, hold a dumbbell in your desired weight lengthwise in front of your chest with elbows loose. While keeping your hips and knees facing forward, twist your torso to the side. To do this move effectively you must be sitting as straight as possible. Make sure your abs are contracting. This move works your abdominal muscles and oblique muscles.

Doing this routine for 3 times per week for 6 weeks will show increased muscle strength and definition. After 6 weeks you should increase your dumbbell weight. 5 pounds for all moves requiring a dumbbell is the recommended increase. For moves that use your body as resistance, such as squats and lunges, you can increase your moves by 12 each week. This will keep you challenged. The thing about body weight bearing exercise is that your body rarely gets sick of them. They are always beneficial and toning, assuming that you do more each time it gets a little too easy.

Play Games with Your Children
If you have children, playing with them outside can be hugely effective for weight loss. Studies show that those that "play"

usually have better health, happiness, and body weights. Playing sports with your children is great quality family time but also burns a lot of calories. Here are some ideas for playing with your children outdoors:

- Ride bikes together.

- Play soccer.

- Go to the park and swing on the swing sets.

- Play catch.

- Take them to the gym with you as your workout buddy.

- Go for a hike.

- Go for a walk and play games while walking, such as I Spy.

- Play volleyball.

- Play fetch with your dog if you have one.

- Go swimming in the summer.

3.3 - Ineffective Exercise

Exercises That Do Not Benefit Weight Loss
It may seem shocking to read that there are exercises that do not help with weight loss. Any type of movement is great for your overall health, but not necessarily for losing weight. As a whole most Americans overestimate the amount of calories they burn and the effort they put in for their workouts. This

can be a big problem, because even if you are exercising you may be consuming extra calories because you thought you burned 400 calories but you only burned 150.

For this reason, any exercise that does not raise your heart rate to at least 130 beats per minute, is going to be a waste of time in terms of weight loss. Even low-impact exercise will often raise your heart rate to 130 or more, including yoga and Pilates. Very slow walks are not considered exercise for weight loss, and if you cannot maintain intensity swimming then that should be avoided as well.

Exercises That Can Hurt Your Physical Well-Being

Any exercise that is out of your league will result in injury. This is particularly true for those that try to push themselves too hard without the help of a professional. For this reason you should be careful whenever you embark upon a new exercise, and if you feel pain then you must stop immediately.

Running, if you are prepared for it, will be a fantastic new fitness routine. But if you are not ready for the intensity and demanding nature of running, then do not try to run. This can hurt your physical health and make it so that you are unable to exercise for a period of time. Common injuries include lower back damages, ankle sprains, foot damage, and knee pain.

Intense boot camp routines are a fantastic way to get in toned and sweat off calories, but again, it can hurt you more than help if you are not prepared. For this reason, avoid any boot camp classes, DVDs, or routines at the start of your weight loss program. After 2 or 3 months of consistent exercises, you should be able to attend a boot camp class without any difficulty or injuries.

Rock climbing and other extreme sports are also a generally bad idea. When you engage in these activities without being properly prepared, you put yourself at risk for permanent injury. Even athletes familiar with these types of sports have difficulty completing them without some type of injury.

When you use improper form for weight lifting, it will likely result in a lot of pain and injury. If you feel like a weight is too easy for you, keep using it until you are sure you can move up a notch. You should be able to just barely finish your reps with your muscles burning. Jumping right to lifting 100 pounds is setting you up for disaster.

Overtraining is a serious problem for many people trying to lose weight. While it is often an athlete's problem, overtraining can affect even those that exercise too much. Doing any amount of physical activity for too many hours without proper rest between days, can result in exhaustion. You begin to feel run down, cranky, constantly hungry, and you stop seeing results.

Why does this happen? When the body isn't allowed to rest for adequate periods of time, it keeps going. When you are forced to run on no energy or proper rest, muscles and joints become fatigued. This fatigue can slow metabolism, decrease the happy mood exercise provides, and lead to a weight rebound.

It's great to be excited about weight loss and exercise, but doing too much is never a good thing. Limit yourself to a maximum of one hour of exercise every day, or two hours of exercise a day with two days of rest. If you are doing high intensity exercise, one hour is sufficient in the beginning. You can work up to two full hours of intense exercise later on with the advice of a medical professional.

Sweat suits are also a very scary trend used by those trying to lose weight. These are plastic-like suits that are designed to make you sweat profusely while walking, running, or weight lifting. People believe that extra sweating will result in more weight loss and detoxing. Sweat suits are extremely dangerous and should not be used. Using these garments will cause dehydration, fainting, heat exhaustion, illness, and muscle fatigue. Your body can go into shock if you pair a sweat suit with any of the exercises listed above, as well as something simple, such as walking. Even if you are drinking plenty of water while wearing one, you are defeating the purpose of using it in the first place. Sweat suits should be avoided at all costs.

Exercises That Can Exacerbate Current Physical Conditions

Exercise is a cure-all for medical conditions and overall health, but there are simply some things you should not do while trying to lose weight. Exercising can heal your body, but only if you do not push yourself into routines that will hurt you even more.

For those with knee problems, avoid running, dancing, or hiking. These put a lot of strain on the knees and causes further weakness of the tendons and muscles. Instead, opt for therapeutic yoga, Pilates, and an elliptical machine. In fact an elliptical machine is a great choice for those with physical conditions because it is low impact.

If you have asthma you may find it hard to do any sort of exercise comfortably. There are many athletes out there that have been able to combat asthma by just working at a slower pace. Anything that makes you breathe at a higher rate than usual is likely to cause an asthma attack. If possible work out in a neutral climate environment with plenty of air filters. This minimizes allergens creeping into your lungs while you exercise. Also take frequent breaks. This can be a challenge if you want to just get your workout over with, but it is worth it to avoid an asthma attack. Walk or use a machine of your choice for 15 minutes, then rest for 5. Repeat until you have completed the number of minutes you desire for your workout routine.

Alternative Exercises for Weight Loss

So you have tried walking and maybe some other equipment at the gym, or you have started a strength training program. You may find that you are getting bored fast, and boredom leads to slacking off when it comes to working out. There are dozens of exercises you can do for weight loss and body toning. All of them will help you reach your goals and give your body a fresh challenge.

Yoga is a very popular and very gentle but effective exercise for weight loss. Incorporating yoga into your workouts on top of your usual routine will result in a calm mind, spirit, body, as well as toned muscles. When someone starts a yoga program they expect it to be easy, but in reality yoga is extremely challenging. If you are worried about taking yoga, then look for different classes or DVDs to suit your needs. There is Bikram yoga, power yoga, weight loss yoga, therapeutic yoga, assisted yoga for those with injury, easy yoga, and much more. Your local instructor should be able to help you find a class to suit your needs.

Zumba is a new fitness craze taking the country by storm. While women usually participate in Zumba, it is for both men and women. This high intensity class mixes dance styles with aerobic exercise. The result is a fast paced Latin inspired workout that burns at least 500 calories per hour. You can expect to burn much more if you weigh more. Zumba will keep things interesting on your days off from your usual cardio routine.

Cycling or Spin Class is a huge favorite amongst gym goers. Easily tailored to suit your workout needs, Cycling can be a challenging but fun exercise. It also torches upwards of 800 calories depending on the class. With an engaging environment and upbeat music, you will stay engaged through the full 30 to 60 minutes. Cycling is safe and relatively low impact. Your legs do a lot of the work but the motion is gentle on the knees. Seats on spin bikes are also very comfortable, unlike most traditional bicycles.

Kettlebell workouts are a bit more advanced than your average weight training routine. However, they are effective at working multiple groups of muscles and burning a significant amount of calories during and after your workout. Kettlebells come in sizes ranging from 5 pounds to 100 pounds. Lighter bells are recommended for beginners because using the heavier models without proper form can be damaging.

3.4 - Fitness Challenges
Starting a fitness challenge at the beginning of your journey is the best way to determine where you stand. A good fitness

challenge is one that tests various different actions and determines how long you can hold those positions or moves. In some instances it is based on how many of an exercise you complete before becoming absolutely exhausted.

A physical fitness level assessment is important because you will know what you need to improve and the route to take for all of your exercise needs. Assessments are a lot like those things that everyone had to do in High School Physical Education. In other words, they are unpleasant but necessary.

For a good fitness indicator test you should:

Hold plank pose for as long as you can. One minute is considered ideal.

Do as many pushups as possible. Less than 10 is considered unsatisfactory. You should aim for at least 10 pushups.

The mile test is where you walk one mile as fast as you can without overexerting yourself. Less than 18 minutes is great, while more than that is unsatisfactory and needs improvement.

The stretch test which measures how far you can stretch is also important. Sit and reach is important, however simple it is. The further you can reach the more flexible you are. If you cannot reach your toes in a seated legs forward position, then try to stretch daily to increase your range.

A one minute crunch test will determine how many repetitions can be completed within 1 minute. The higher the score is, the better your fitness level.

Simple fitness assessments can be done at home as long as you have someone watching you and counting for your repetitions. You can also go to a local gym and ask for a trainer to help you with a fitness assessment, but be warned that you may have to pay fees. Some gyms offer this for free.

3.5 - Sports Wear Accessories to Add To Your Routine

Adding equipment is completely optional but some people may find them to be very beneficial for their weight loss program. There are hundreds of products out there that claim to boost weight loss and help you shed pounds faster, but you don't need all of them. Even adding a few new things to your exercise and weight loss plan can boost your results.

The BodyBugg

This device was originally used by professionals to monitor laboratory weight loss efforts. Since then the BodyBugg has been used on top television weight loss shows like "The Biggest Loser." This device is worn for 24 hours a day, 7 days a week. It keeps track of how much you burn the entire day, so that you know how much to eat. This device costs about $250 including 6 months of their required online program, but sales are frequent. A BodyBugg is recommended for those with a lot of weight to lose.

http://bodybugg.com/

A Weighted Vest

If your normal routine is becoming too easy, add in a weighted vest. They come in weights from 10 pounds to 75 pounds and up. Weighted vests will strengthen your core muscles while walking or running, as well as provide more resistance and calorie burn. This is recommended for individuals that have lost weight already and are stronger than they were at the start of a program.

Nordic Walking Poles

Adding walking poles may seem like it would reduce the efficiency of exercise, but they actually increase calorie burn by up to 40%. Walking poles help you balance but also keep your arms engaged in movement. They are also good for stabilizing on rocky surfaces, such as during a hike. Walking poles are useful for a lot of things when exercising outdoors, and should be part of every walker's routine. Poles can range from $15 to $150 for a set.

Quality Shoes

Having quality shoes cannot be stressed enough. While they do not promote weight loss on their own, they do protect your ankles, knees, and feet. Having stable shoes for your terrain of choice is extremely important. Good running or walking shoes are a must, but if you hike on rugged ground then you will want to purchase hiking or trail shoes.

Weighted Ankle and Wrist Weights

These usually come in small weight amounts but add a big impact to your workout. Try swinging your arms back and forth while wearing 2 pound weights on each arm. Or take a fitness class with ankle and wrist weights. These strengthen the muscles in those areas that are often difficult to train, so you burn more calories while gaining hard to build muscle in the wrists and ankles.

Bosu Ball

The bosu ball is an interesting device that resembles a half ball with a solid plastic base. These look simple and useless, but the core training they provide is astounding. Bosu balls are expensive and usually cost $60 to $100 for one. But standing on them will challenge your balance and core muscles. You can do pushups on them, crunches, planks, and many more. Bosu balls support a lot of weight too, so you do not need to worry about them popping or bursting while performing exercises.

Comfortable Pants and T-Shirts

It sounds weird, but having comfortable and slightly loose workout clothes will help you perform better. Being constricted in jeans and fitted tops will make exercising awkward and uncomfortable. Additionally, most fitness centers do not permit them.

At-Home Equipment

If you have money and space, invest in at home fitness equipment. An elliptical or treadmill makes a great at-home gym for days when you can't make it to a real gym. Or even if you prefer to workout at home, you can do so without feeling uncomfortable. Home equipment is more affordable than it was in the past, and ideal for those with limited time to go elsewhere for their fitness needs.

4 - Accomplishing your Weight Loss Goals

Weight loss goals are the entire reason anyone wants to lose weight and get healthy for good. Keeping your goals in mind will be the foundation of your effort. Without any idea on what goals you want, you will be stuck without guidance and end up failing. Setting goals is as important as accomplishing them. As you accomplish those goals you feel a sense of strength and power from overcoming your self doubts.

Keeping Realistic Goals

Losing weight is never easy. It takes time, dedication, and effort every single day. When you set your weight loss goals you should keep several factors in mind. What do you want to lose overall? What do you hope to accomplish in the long run? How will these changes benefit your lifestyle? Having comprehensive solid goals in sight will help you along the way. Fad diets and national media promote ridiculous goals that are full of promises that are unobtainable. Losing 15 pounds in 2 weeks is not healthy, nor is it feasible to keep that weight off for any significant period of time. Fast diets and crazy tactics will not only make you sick, but they will make you fatter than you were to begin with.

For realistic purposes, the BMI chart is not going to help you. It states that a 5 foot 4 inch tall female should weigh about 125 pounds. For women and men that have been overweight for years or most of their lives, these numbers can be daunting and unrealistic. The important thing to consider is your body fat percentage, how you feel, and muscle strength. Developing these things instead of reaching a very small number will be better for your health. Additionally, the BMI should only be a rough example, not an indicator of true health or progress or what goals you should aim for.

Write Down Your Goals

You can type them online but physically writing them makes your brain think they are more significant. You remember things better if you write with a pen and paper. So write down what you want to accomplish in 1 month, 3 months, 6 months, 1 year, and 5 years. It takes time to make a permanent lifestyle change.

Fill out a sheet, print it, and hang it somewhere to read everyday. Post notes where you will see them the most. Writing down these goals will keep them fresh in your mind. The reason people have setbacks is because they don't keep their goals and desires "fresh." It's difficult to have these thoughts in your head every minute, but it is one of the only ways to make things a habit, and thus reach your final goal point.

Visualize Your Goals

How do you visualize your goals? Make a collage or post inspirational photos and clippings on your fridge. Having something positive to look at while you prepare meals or look for food in the freezer will make a huge impact on how you stick to your meal plan. Constantly imagine yourself at your desired weight. Imagine your strong muscles or lean limbs. Imagine excess visceral fat fleeing your body to allow your organs room to operate at full power. Imagine your arteries clearing up and pumping blood to your heart without any strain. These are significant changes that will make you feel good about sticking to a diet and weight loss plan.

Visualization may even be powerful for helping you shed a few extra pounds too. Try to meditate daily and imagine yourself healthier and stronger. Meditation is proven to boost mood and make difficult habits easier to break.

Yoga is an excellent exercise for helping you to visualize your goals. When you twist into positions and are forced to meditate and relax, your body does amazing things. Constant visualization is one of the top ways to keep going in the right direction.

Pick Yourself Up

If you fall off track, pick yourself up and start again. If you fall off track for a few weeks, start over. The goal is to never stop trying to improve your healthy lifestyle. One day of overeating is not the end of the world, but you should recognize the mistakes you made. When you realize that eating a 2,000 calorie meal in one sitting doesn't make you feel so great, you will think twice about doing it again in the future. It must be stressed frequently that losing weight does not happen overnight. One mistake can set you back for the week, but it will not set you back forever.

Aim For the 10% Goal

Most people set extraordinarily high standards for how much weight they want to lose. If you weigh 200 pounds, losing 30% of your total body weight would be astounding. But 10% alone is enough for you to see significant health changes. 10% is all it takes. That's only 20 pounds if you weigh 200 pounds. This can be achieved faster than a 50 or 60 pounds goal. Keep 10% in your head and you will be successful.

Starting Small Leads to Something Big

When you are told to start small, it isn't a joke. Don't smirk or roll your eyes. Don't think you can lose 30 pounds in a single month or bench press 200 pounds immediately. Jumping into something and moving much faster than you are will set you up for injury, disappointment, and a loss of your overall goal. Starting small however, will make you feel proud of the little accomplishments. You will work up to running 2 miles per workout. You will work up to lifting 200 pounds. You can even work up to running a marathon one day. Everything is possible, as long as you start small and keep your goals organized.

Having an action plan for reaching the big things is a great way to get there faster. There are few things more satisfying than doing something big once you have improved yourself and pushed your body to the limits.

Dealing with Setbacks

A setback is bound to happen. Most people that have lost astounding amounts of weight have been set back several times. As the old proverb says, "Fall down seven times, stand up eight." If you get stuck and can't lose weight, keep pushing. Change your routine, tweak your calorie consumption. You will get over the setbacks and shed weight again. If you reach a setback, re-evaluate your goals. They may be too difficult for your lifestyle or not suited for your body type. Re-evaluation is all right, and you are not admitting defeat if you have to do this.

If anything, the event of having a setback should be motivation to try harder towards accomplishing your goal. Ask for advice from a professional and remember not to skip meals or forget to stay hydrated or else your body can actually try to hold onto extra weight as a survival strategy. Whatever you choose to do, you need to make sure that you do not stop in your efforts for healthy weight loss.

Measure Your Progress

Most people hop on the scale and measure their progress based on how much they weigh. Weight measurement is fine and it should be done on a regular basis. But for a number of reasons, your weight is not the most accurate identifier of the true progress your body has made.

At the beginning of your weight loss journey, measure the following body areas:

- Hips

- Waist (around the belly button)

- Chest

- Neck

- Bicep

- Thigh

These are the most important areas to track, as people tend to lose fat from them frequently. Your waist is especially important to measure for progress. Fat in the waist is the most dangerous kind of fat there is. Losing inches in your waist is more beneficial than shedding pounds overall. But chances are if you are losing fat there you will be losing pounds all over. Measurements are important because you can gauge if you are changing shape and size. You can weigh 20 pounds less but if you aren't changing actual size that can be disappointing. If you plateau you can take measurements to see if something else has changed.

Measuring body fat percentage is also a way to gauge your progress. It is ideal to get your body fat measured by a professional fitness trainer. He or she can measure your fat accurately once per month. This will show that even if you aren't losing number weight on the scale, your percentage of body fat is likely to be going down.

You can also revisit fitness assessments to determine your progress physically. These should be done every 2 months to see if your strength and efficiency is improving. Having better physical health is a fantastic motivator.

Find A Weight Loss Partner Or Gym Buddy
Usually when you tell your friends and family about a new weight loss plan, they will look at you with doubt. It's difficult

to deal with close friends telling you all the negative things about your diet, even if you are following just a general diet plan of eating healthier and eating less junk food. It seems like those closest to you want to see you fail. Having a weight loss partner and or gym buddy can be a great way to stay focused and accountable for what you consume.

If any of your friends are trying a new healthy lifestyle program, ask if they would like to be your buddy. Keep each other in check and have healthy lunches together in your free time. When you have someone by your side it is easier to accomplish your goals.

A gym buddy is also a great way to keep you going after the first 10 minutes of a tough workout. Take classes together at the gym and talk to each other on the treadmill. Having a support system will keep you going even when you are doubting yourself. If a friend is counting on you to show up at the gym, you are more likely to follow through and just go.

If you don't know anyone locally you can probably find a buddy online. There are countless sources for finding an online workout buddy, which can be just as effective. You can text each other, email, or IM to hold yourselves accountable. You could share pictures of your healthy meals and tips about how your day went.

A strong support system is vital, but telling your entire family and friends circle is a bad idea. Most will try to sabotage your efforts. During get-togethers don't make a point to say you can't eat certain foods. Just ignore those foods or take a very small portion.

Sticking With Your Plan For The Long Haul

Once you commit to a lifestyle change it is vital to stick with your plan. A yo-yo effect of eating healthy then eating junk food is not only bad for your health but bad for your psyche too. Many people get stuck on being perfect 24/7, but the reality is that being perfect isn't possible. There will be days where you choose to eat a slice of cake. That's OK every once in awhile; your body will appreciate treats. The problem is when you eat a sweet treat daily.

Sticking with your plan for as long as you can is important. That is why health gurus and doctors push the idea of a lifestyle change. With a lifestyle change, being healthy becomes habit. You learn to read labels and count calories without thinking too hard. Eating 8 servings of fruits and vegetables per day becomes second nature.

Diet fads do not encourage a lifestyle change that is manageable. Between counting carbohydrates and following crazy week by week plans, these diets are stressful and complicated. They are not maintainable over a long period of time. They may work for a month or two, but when it comes to keeping the weight off permanently, you will be at a loss to keep up.

Using online tools to your advantage will also help you stay on track. Join a community where you can discuss your frustrations, ask for tips and keep track of your food. Most people are friendly and will answer whatever questions you have to the best of their ability. Losing weight in the modern world is easier than ever, especially with technology on your side. There are countless apps and programs to literally shout out exercises for you to do throughout the day. There are on-the-go applications that give you nutrition information at fast food restaurants and other eating establishments.

With all of these gadgets available, losing weight and sticking to your plan will be a fun journey that is full of rewards and good health. Once you lose that first 10% of your goal you will be motivated to keep going. You will not want to stop and go back to your old unhealthy ways. Change doesn't happen overnight, but you can make your goals a reality by starting today.

4.1 - Maintaining Your Progress

Once you have reached your goal, you will feel amazing, accomplished, and stronger than ever. Losing weight of any amount is a huge accomplishment that should not be taken lightly. After you reach your goal though, you will still need to maintain your healthy lifestyle change.

Eating healthy will be an important step to follow the rest of your life. If you find yourself slipping into old habits, simply recheck yourself and remember that you never want to return to your old ways. This is why diets rarely work. Once someone stops a diet they go back to their old ways. Learning a healthy lifestyle change is a permanent solution that will help you live a long and healthy life. Reaching your ultimate goal can take time, but with perseverance you will reach those numbers.

Once you reach your goal you will need to do one of two things:

1. Maintain your goal

2. Strive for something better

Maintaining your goal weight may seem like an easy task but once you have reached your goal you will need to really keep a strategy for yourself to reduce the chances of weight gain in recoil. Most people think that once you are at your goal weight that it is now acceptable to stop your exercise regimen. The truth of the matter is that you will still need to work out on a schedule and continue to plan your diet so that your body maintains a healthy metabolism. If you stop cold turkey at any point you will risk:

A metabolism rate slow down - This will cause your body to reduce its efficiency in processing what you eat into immediate energy and will instead focus more on energy storage as fats for future use. A slow metabolism will also reduce energy levels when you decide to eat which can cause problems after eating larger meals.

A reduction in elasticity – Your body does not maintain your ability to stretch out and stay flexible without working for it. By reducing your body motion and exercise your muscles and tendons will tighten up slowly over time. The next time you decide to become active after a long period of rest may bring you back to a previous state of elasticity, even if you have not gained any weight. It will take time to regain your elasticity.

Rapid weight gain – If your diet goes off track and back into consuming larger amounts of calories while staying sedentary, your body will begin to revert back into a slow metabolism rate which will increase storage of fats. Weight gain can occur at a rapid pace when the body becomes less active.

Increased Fatigue – By not maintaining your progress, your body will be placed on a higher load to process what you eat.

This will cause your body to take more energy to do things like digest the food you ingest while increasing the need for the liver to create bile to process fats and the pancreas to create more insulin to process sugars and carbohydrates. Other organs are also working hard to maintain balance in your body. All of this extra stress is very taxing on the body which will lead to fatigue and a feeling of lethargy.

Reduced Libido – Once the body has been inactive and has begun to regain weight, the sex drive may decrease substantially. This is not the only factor in reduced libido that can become a problem. Not having proper exercise can make it difficult to keep a pace during physical relations. This could also lead to problems for both men and women by not allowing them to climax properly.

By taking the simple routine of maintenance for your weight loss goal, you can ensure that these problems do not make their way into your now healthier life. Maintaining your goal weight is possible by taking advantage of the practices that you have put in place for weight loss. Of course, you do not need to be as strict with your maintenance to remain in your goal weight but it is beneficial to stick to it as much as possible.

Setting new goals once you have reached your original weight loss goal is also a great way to get into even better shape. Instead of focusing on weight loss, you can try taking the route of muscle building or toning your existing mass. You can even set a goal to lose more weight, if you still have weight to lose. Setting a new goal will make it possible for you to keep yourself working towards better health.

While you are making your healthy lifestyle changes, you occasionally have to have some fun or find information that helps you as well as others along that path. The following sites are some that can lead to do just that: get involved in life.

Just for a bit of fun, take a good friend or your partner to an entertaining event in your area. You can find the shows and concerts you are interested in at http://www.econcertticketsforsale.com/ . Sometimes a bit of culture shared is a benefit in getting to know the people around you.

For even more fun, you can try Pro Flight Simulator to experience your own adventure. You can find more information at http://www.proflightsimulator101.com/ and build your own excitement in the comfort of your own home.

If you are more of an outdoor type of person, you can find information on camping tents and trailers at http://tentsandmoreonline.com/ to find what suits your tastes. Sometimes a quiet night under the stars is what gives you a chance to reflect on life and continue to find your path.

For the ladies that are not blessed with long, luxurious eyelashes, cosmetics can add to your beauty and boost your self-esteem during your weight loss process. One product that comes highly recommended can be found at http://idollash.co/.

When you decide to settle down in life, children are usually brought to mind. Moms-to-be may find some useful information at http://www.pregnancymiraclesystemx.com/ for before and during their pregnancies. There are times when others in your particular situation help you more than you trying to handle different issues on your own.

These sites are only a sampling to get you started in your exploration of life and in making the changes you want to make. But you will find that there are times that the small distraction of exploring different things will bring you back life and inspire you to stay with your weight loss plan.